"As a seasoned psychoanalyst w___ g___ ___p___ ___ ___

matters, Dr. Savelle-Rocklin enables readers to understand, and master, the real causes of their compulsive eating. By looking beyond the surface of *what* you eat to *why* you eat, she brings clarity to this very misunderstood area."

—**Lance Dodes, MD**, assistant clinical professor of psychiatry (retired), Harvard Medical School; author of *The Heart of Addiction, Breaking Addiction*, and *The Sober Truth*

"*The Binge Cure* outlines practical tips and techniques to make peace with food and your body. Dr. Nina Savelle-Rocklin is a renowned expert on the issue and provides critical insight to overcome emotional overeating, stop dieting, and live the physically and emotionally healthy life that you deserve!"

—**Jacquelyn Ekern, MS, LPC**, president at Weight Hope, Addiction Hope, and Eating Disorder Hope

"Listeners to Dr. Nina's weekly program on L.A. Talk Radio know that she focuses on what's eating 'at' you instead of on what you're eating. In this book she brings wisdom, knowledge, and compassion to help readers understand and change their emotional eating habits. *The Binge Cure* is a must-read for anyone who craves a healthier, happier relationship to themselves."

—**Craig Ramsay**, celebrity trainer and fitness expert, author of *Anatomy of Stretching*

"Dr. Nina hits an emotional bull's-eye zeroing in on the unmistakable truth behind the reality of binge eating and its successful treatment in *The Binge Cure*. This game-changing book provides a road map to assist readers in identifying the pain that fuels the fury of so-called food addiction and learning to recognize the relationship between the foods one reaches for and the circumstances under which they're reaching. Full of exercises that accompany case examples of patients from her thriving private practice—patients who have achieved success utilizing her methods—Dr. Nina provides a much-needed solution to the epidemic of eating disorders that are consuming society. Brilliantly written with the compassionate voice of someone who has triumphed in the battlefield herself, *The Binge Cure* provides the truth of why diets will never work and arms the reader with the knowledge necessary to successfully navigate that pain and rise above it."

—**Kelley Gunter**, author of *You Have Such a Pretty Face*

"This book is THE BIBLE on how to pry yourself off the scale and out of the never-ending cycle of yo-yo dieting, food obsession, and confusing your life goals with your weight goals. Dr. Nina tackles the tough questions and the complicated issues surrounding food, emotional eating, and physical well-being. And her solutions are sensible and based on real case studies, her guidance indispensable. This book is a keeper."

—**Iris Ruth Pastor**, author of *The Secret Life of a Weight-Obsessed Woman: Wisdom to Live the Life You Crave*

THE BINGE CURE

*7 Steps to Outsmart
Emotional Eating*

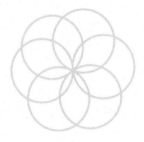

NINA SAVELLE-ROCKLIN, PsyD

ADLER PRESS

Library of Congress Control Number: 2019904826

© 2019 Nina Savelle-Rocklin, PsyD

Cover and text design: Diana Nuhn

The material in this book is intended to provide accurate and authoritative information but should not be used as a substitute for professional care. The author and publisher urge you to consult with your mental health care provider or seek other professional advice in the event that you require expert assistance.

For my loves,
David, Ariel, and Kavanna.
And, of course, Zane.

CONTENTS

PREFACE

How often do you lose control over food? Maybe you wake up every morning with the best intentions. You vow to be "good" and stick to your diet. Over the next several days or weeks, you eat right, go to the gym, and drop a few pounds. Maybe you get your hopes up that this is finally it. You dream of slipping on a pair of skinny jeans, imagining sliding them over your hips with ease.

Before you know it, you fall off the diet wagon by eating one of your forbidden foods. To cope with the feelings of guilt, you polish off the rest of that dessert, pizza, bag of chips, or whatever you were eating. When it's time to get back on track, there are so many choices: Weight Watchers, Paleo, Whole30, South Beach, Mediterranean, low-carb, high-carb, liquid diet, cookie diet, and ketogenic. You start another diet only to get derailed again and gain back the weight you just lost.

Maybe you also try counting steps as well as calories, but you wind up with a really cool Fitbit and zero sustainable weight loss. So there you are with two different sets of clothes in your closet— one for the size you are and one for the size you want to be. You're more than ready for something new, but you don't know what to do instead of dieting. You're afraid that if you're not on some kind of diet, you're going to pack on the pounds. You're afraid you're always going to look like a "before" photo. That fit, slim "after" photo seems like an impossible dream.

Here's the good news: In this book, I'm going to show you exactly how to create permanent, sustainable weight loss. No dieting necessary. Not only will you finally be able to fit into those skinny jeans in the back of your closet, but you'll also break free from your preoccupation with food and dieting. For so many dieters, the goal isn't just changing the number on the scale. You want to stop the obsession with food, to stop thinking about every bite.

As a psychoanalyst specializing in food, weight, and body image issues, I'm here to help you navigate a path to lasting weight loss without counting calories, fat grams, or carbs. You may be wondering what exactly a psychoanalyst does and how that differs from other kinds of therapy. One of my patients said it best: "Therapy is like snorkeling. You go a little bit under the surface and see some cool things. But analysis? That's like deep-sea diving to the bottom of the ocean. It's pitch black and you've got to shine a light in the darkness to see what's down there."

Shining that light helps you discover the hidden reasons that you're turning to food. In my private clinical practice and through my online programs, I've helped thousands of people all over the world heal their relationship with food, stop bingeing, lose weight, and gain health. In this book I will give you powerful strategies to achieve your goals, using the exact steps I use with my private clients.

My work is highly personal and important to me. Early in my career I created a support group for women who were struggling with binge eating. At the time I was interning at a local counseling center. The staff took care of the entire intake process, interviewing prospective group members and deciding who was a good candidate. That meant that I didn't meet any of the group members until our first session. I spent many hours getting ready for that group. This was my first experience as a group facilitator, and I was determined to give these women a mind-opening, body-changing, soul-shifting transformation.

On the day of the first group meeting, I swung open the door to the therapy room. Eight women sat on the overstuffed chairs and slightly worn couch, each of them looking uncomfortable and a bit nervous. Their ages ranged from twenties to fifties. A few carried an extra ten or twenty pounds. Others were a hundred pounds overweight.

"Hi there," I said, entering the room.

A redhead in her late fifties, wearing a brightly colored shirt and a necklace with huge, colorful beads, fixed her gaze on me. Her body overflowed her chair, and her mouth was a tight line on her face.

She said, *"You're* the therapist? Seriously?"

I tried to keep the smile on my face. The group hadn't even started, and somehow I'd already disappointed this woman. I tried to figure out the problem. Was she expecting someone older? Someone with more experience? Was it totally obvious that this was my first group?

"Yes, I'm the therapist," I repeated, hoping that my voice didn't sound as unsteady as it felt. I checked the roster of names on my clipboard. "And you are . . . ?"

"My name's Carole. So, what does a skinny bitch like you know about binge eating?"

The room was quiet. Then it got even quieter. My heart was pounding. I couldn't believe this was happening. Did she really just call me a *skinny bitch*?

The others shifted awkwardly, avoiding my gaze. At that moment I had an epiphany. I realized when they looked at me, they didn't see someone who understood them. Someone who could identify with their pain. Who could relate to their challenges and anxieties.

"I know a lot, actually," I said, taking a seat.

Carole crossed her arms, looking skeptical.

"Let me put it this way," I indicated myself with a wave of a hand. "This skinny bitch once ate an entire bag of gingerbread cookies in about fifteen minutes flat."

I had their attention. I added, "And I hate gingerbread."

I felt the tension easing. The women looked at me with curiosity. "My eating problems go back to when I was five years old," I told them. "I remember the exact moment I decided that my thighs were too big. I never looked at magazines or watched TV, so I had no media influences. Still, I was positive that if my legs were thinner, I'd somehow be better. And I was a perfectly normal-weight kid."

My obsession grew worse as I got older. Every page of every one of my journals was filled with numbers. I wrote down what I ate, what I didn't eat, how much I weighed, and how much I was going to weigh after the next diet. I fell asleep counting calories and fat grams, wondering if I'd lose weight the next morning or gain it.

When I hiked with friends, I wasn't focusing on the beautiful day. I wasn't actually enjoying time with my friends. Instead of connecting with them, I was focused on how many calories I was burning. I was always on some crazy diet that was usually extremely restrictive. Eventually my willpower failed and I would binge and then take laxatives or use other measures so I wouldn't gain weight.

I finally went to therapy. But I went for anxiety, not for my eating problems. I shared my boyfriend issues, my goals, my dreams, and my fears. I was open with my therapist about every aspect of my life—except one. I never told her what was going on with food. I was too ashamed to admit the truth.

In the months that followed, I began noticing small changes. I stopped counting calories instead of sheep to fall asleep. I started paying more attention to my feelings. When I got upset I stopped getting frustrated with myself. I became a friend to myself instead of a critic. Those crazy binge episodes began occurring less frequently. Eventually I completely stopped using food to cope. By the time I left treatment, all of my destructive food behaviors had disappeared. Interestingly, not once—not a single time—did I ever tell my therapist about my horrible relationship with food.

How was this possible? After all, I was a self-described poster child for eating disorders. How in the world did I liberate myself from a continuous cycle of dieting and bingeing without ever talking about food? Simple. My behavior was a solution to the real problem, which was my toxic relationship with myself. When I made peace with myself, I made peace with food too.

I finished my story and looked into the gaze of the group members. For several horrible seconds I regretted what I had said. Had my self-disclosure made things worse? Was I a bad therapist? Did these women hate me?

Carol said, "You were only five years old. Why in the world did you think your thighs were big?"

I told her that as a child I was considered "too much" to handle. My parents, who were college professors, were intellectual and academic. Their idea of spending family time was visiting the library on a Sunday morning. We scattered to different parts of the library to find books. Afterward we went home and read those books in different rooms.

Reading wasn't my idea of a good time—I was more spirited and energetic. My family told me that I was too loud, too sensitive, too dramatic, and too emotional. The overall message was that I was "too much" to handle. My five-year-old mind translated this as being literally too much, too big. My issues with food and body image reflected a wish to be smaller and somehow more acceptable.

Carole said, "I hate it when people assume things about me just because I'm fat." She took a moment and heaved a sigh. "I hate to admit this, but that's what I did to you. I made assumptions because you're thin."

Another woman spoke up. "That happens to me every day. People assume I'm lazy, greedy, or have no willpower."

"Me too," said someone else.

And just like that, the group found common ground. We started talking about what it was like to be judged by our appearance. One woman shared the humiliating experience of asking a flight attendant for a seat-belt extension. Another cringed as she recalled the judgmental looks from shoppers at the grocery store as they passed her shopping cart, which was filled with boxes of cookies and ice cream. A mother tearfully talked about the time her tween daughter shared how embarrassed she was to have an overweight mother.

That bonding moment lasted through the rest of our time together. Carole scared the heck out of me at first, but ultimately she taught me an important lesson about vulnerability. Instead of being "the therapist" and positioning myself as an expert, I realized I had to trust my humanity and share that part of myself with my patients.

The artist Michelangelo created some of the world's most beautiful art, including the iconic statues of David, *Madonna of Bruges*, and countless other pieces. Someone asked Michelangelo how he turned those great blocks of stone into statues.

"Every block of stone has a statue inside it, and it is the task of the sculptor to discover it."

I love this story because it's a perfect description of change. People who struggle with food often describe themselves as "broken" and think there's something wrong with them. They aren't broken. They're just stuck. Our work together is always to chip away at what keeps them stuck, so that they can be their most genuine and true selves.

It's never too late to change. I've helped men and women from their early teens to their late seventies transform their relationship with food. No matter what life stage you are in, no matter what you've endured, no matter how hopeless you think your situation may seem, there is always hope. It really is possible to free yourself from your fixation with food and to enjoy your life.

As one of the clients in my online program wrote, "Thank you for freeing me from forty years of dieting and living on low-fat foods and sugar-free this and that. I'm in Paris and enjoying some tasty French food, with no inner critic bullying me. Here's to freedom and living life to the max!"

If you want to experience that kind of freedom, keep reading.

INTRODUCTION

Let me be very clear: This is not a diet book. You won't have to keep track of food or count calories, carbs, or anything else. You won't find nutritional advice in any of the following chapters. If that's what you're looking for, then stop reading. This isn't the book for you.

What you will find is a way to stop binge eating, to lose the obsession and preoccupation with every bite. You'll discover a way to lose weight and keep it off for good. If you're sick and tired of dieting, this book offers a solution. By following the steps outlined in the following chapters, you will experience what thousands of people in my private practice and online program have experienced: liberation.

It really is possible to free yourself from a lifetime of dieting and see results. My patient, whom I'll call Alyssa (all names of patients in this book have been changed for confidentiality reasons), is a good example of this. Alyssa stopped bingeing, lost weight, and kept it off, without ever counting a single calorie, carb, or fat gram. At first she was skeptical about my approach, which was different from anything she had tried before. During our initial consultation, she told me she'd tried everything—every diet, every workout, everything short of surgery. She figured she had nothing to lose by giving my non-dieting approach a try.

That first session took place on a hot, sticky, and uncomfortable summer day. Alyssa showed up wearing dark jeans and a long-sleeved sweatshirt.

She said, "I thought about wearing shorts. Honestly, I'd rather have heatstroke than let anyone see my legs."

Alyssa chose camouflage over comfort, dressing to hide her body from others. She worried about her health as well as her appearance, and often struggled with depression and anxiety about her weight. She feared her situation was hopeless and that no one could help her.

"I feel so stuck," she said. "Every other part of my life is pretty good, but my binge eating keeps getting worse. I can't believe how much weight I've gained. How do I get over this terrible eating problem?"

> "I can assure you with absolute certainty that you do not have an eating problem."

If you're reading this book, you may think you have an eating problem, or you know someone who does. I can assure you with absolute certainty that you do not have an eating problem. This may sound controversial, but, in fact, there is no such thing as an eating problem.

Weight-loss diets focus on *what* you're eating but not *why*. Diets don't address the underlying reasons you turn to food in the first place. Imagine you have a garden in your backyard. Every day you visit that garden and see that weeds have popped up among your plants and flowers. You pull out the weeds, but what happens when you don't get the roots? Your garden looks great for a little while, and then . . . the weeds grow back! And you have to start all over.

Diets are like weeds. You've likely pulled out weed after weed to resolve your weight problems. For a while it probably worked; you lost weight and started to feel better. And then you found yourself right back where you started—bingeing, dieting, and obsessing in front of the mirror. You feel out of control and you hate the way you look. Here's where you must have compassion for yourself and understand why it has been hard to create lasting change. After all, you can't solve a problem you don't see.

The reason you're still struggling is this: You haven't gotten to the root of why you eat, binge, or constantly diet. You haven't accessed these parts because you didn't know they were there. Those roots are outside of your awareness, deep in your unconscious, hidden from you.

The key to permanent change is finding those roots and pulling them out. That's where I can help you. In this book I will teach you how to look inside of yourself and identify your binge triggers, and then I'll show you how to make sustainable, permanent changes.

Getting back to Alyssa, her main problem was that she could not stop bingeing at night. She was busy all day, and her relationship with food was okay. Nights were a completely different story. She ate a normal dinner and then, even though she wasn't hungry, she always found herself snacking after dinner. She kept eating even when she was so full that her stomach hurt.

I helped Alyssa realize that this was a way of converting emotional pain to physical pain. While she was at work, she wasn't thinking about what was bothering her. When she was home with her thoughts, she felt restless and upset, so she turned to food. She had no idea how to soothe herself without food. When she identified and worked through what was bothering her, she stopped bingeing and lost weight. I'll tell you more about how she did that in just a little while.

One way of getting rid of those underlying conflicts is to be in psychoanalysis or analytic psychotherapy. In today's fast-paced and hectic world, many people don't have the time or resources to commit to such an undertaking, nor does everyone have access to psychoanalytic treatment. I wrote this book so you can manage this problem yourself. Like Alyssa, you really can stop bingeing, lose weight, and gain health, all without ever going on another diet.

In the first chapter of the book, we'll dig into the science and psychology of why diets actually make you gain weight. The truth is, dieting is bad for your health. Body positivity activist Taryn Brumfitt says, "I never trust a four-letter word where the first three letters spell 'die.'" Diets destroy your ability to eat intuitively and compromise your metabolism. Diets kill your mood, spirit, sense of enjoyment, and self-image. When you're on a diet, you're focused on what you should eat (or not eat) instead of listening to your body and eating intuitively. You might be surprised to learn of the growing evidence that diets do more harm than good when it comes to weight loss.

Next we'll crack the code of emotional eating, paying special attention to the hidden emotions and situations that are the biggest triggers. It's impossible to fight an invisible army. As long as what's going on inside remains out of awareness, you just get beaten up by a hidden force and you don't know why. Only by recognizing what's truly taking place inside and making that army visible can you see what's really happening. Then you can fight back—and win.

Like most people, you're probably familiar with the concept of emotional eating. We're going well beyond this concept, but it's our starting point. A huge part of what makes us human is our ability to feel a range of different emotions, yet there are many injunctions against recognizing, sharing, and expressing those feelings. We can't ignore our emotions, can't stuff them down, work them away, gamble them away, or positive-think them away. As counterintuitive as it may seem, the only way to get rid of feelings is to actually express them. I will give you some actionable strategies to do exactly that, which will set the foundation for the rest of the book.

We're also going to launch a counterattack against many of the ideas you have about food. These days it seems that eating is considered almost a criminal act. If you think that seems dramatic, consider these common expressions:

"I was so *bad* last night. I ate pizza."

"I want fried chicken, but I've been so good today, I don't want to ruin it."

"I can't eat dessert in front of my friends. They'll judge me."

Sound familiar? For many of us, eating "bad" foods equates to being bad or feeling bad about ourselves. And the reverse is the idea that eating healthy food means we're being good. Either way, what we eat is connected to our characters. And that's simply not true. Think about it. Your goodness or worthiness isn't tied to what you choose to put in your mouth. Together we're going to change those ideas.

The next step is to make peace with yourself. In this section of the book, you will take back your power from the mirror and the bathroom scale. I'm going to show you how to nurture a healthy relationship with yourself by turning your inner critic into a friend.

You will also get to know your needs. In addition to having basic needs for food, water, and shelter, we all need love, affection, connection, attention, and a sense of purpose or meaningfulness in our lives. If those needs aren't met, or are inconsistently met, we feel "needy." We may turn to food as a way to meet those needs. In this part of the book, we're going to find new ways to respond, other than with food.

Then we're going to look at your relationship to food and to other people. I have a sign in my office that says, "Sometimes when I open my mouth, my mother comes out." Alyssa, for example, was raised by highly critical parents who were never satisfied with her performance in school or in sports. When Alyssa got a report card with five A grades and one B, they scolded her for the B. When she got 100 percent on a test, they wanted to know why she hadn't earned extra credit. When she set a personal record in track, they predicted that she would do even better next time. When she went to a Big 10 college, they were disappointed that she did not attend an Ivy League school. Alyssa wished her parents could appreciate what she did well instead of focusing on what she didn't do.

When Alyssa bought a new home, she immediately criticized herself for not being able to afford a more expensive place. When she made partner at her law firm, she wondered why she hadn't done so earlier. No matter what she accomplished, it was never good enough. As you can see, Alyssa related to the accomplishments and achievements in her current life in exactly the way her parents had during her childhood.

People often ask, "Is it always about the past? Why can't we just deal with what's going on right now?" Our task in this part of the book is to put the past in the past. Just as Alyssa did, when she realized that she was repeating the worst moments of her childhood on a daily basis and instead began to treat herself with more appreciation and respect. And let me be very clear that this isn't about blaming our parents. It's about explaining *why* you learned to cope by eating, in the service of creating something new.

Once you achieve that, the goal is to be fully in the present and find new strategies to relate to yourself. In Alyssa's situation the roots of her relationship with food went deep. She never felt as if she was good enough and had terrible self-esteem. Her lifelong solution to feeling bad was to eat for comfort and then become upset with herself for eating.

Alyssa knew she was a good person but somehow didn't feel *good enough*, and she was sure that other people viewed her the way she saw herself. When she changed her perspective by challenging the assumptions she always took as truisms, she stopped eating for comfort and distraction and lost weight. The last time I saw her, she was wearing a lovely summer dress, no longer trying to hide her legs.

Our minds are incredibly adept at protecting ourselves from unpleasant or upsetting emotions. We often become so good at avoiding what's bothering us that we don't even know we're triggered. If you're turning to food and don't understand why, it's not because you're addicted to food or have no willpower; it's because your mind has found a way to protect you. These modes of protection include turning against yourself, mind reading, slave driving, and minimizing, and we'll explore these behaviors in the book. In this section, we're going to replace eating for distraction with new and effective ways of coping.

If you've ever lost weight and then sabotaged your progress, you're not alone. Lots of people get close to their goal weight and suddenly start making bad food choices or letting their gym memberships lapse. We're going to work together so that when you start losing weight, you stop the sabotage and stay on track. That's when the weight starts coming off naturally and, even more important, remains off.

Keep in mind that change is always a process. No one sits at a piano for the first time and plays a Tchaikovsky concerto right away. First you have to identify the piano keys, learn the chords, and practice. Then you practice some more. You keep practicing until one day you sit down at the piano and play effortlessly. There's a similar sequence to stop bingeing, stop emotional and stress eating, and stop the yo-yo-dieting cycle. Following the steps in this book will help you create a healthier, happier relationship with food for good. You'll stop bingeing, lose weight, gain health, and feel better about yourself than you ever have—all without ever counting a single calorie or fat gram.

Are you ready? Let's get started. . . .

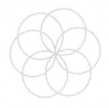

CHAPTER 1

Ditch Dieting

Have you ever noticed how there is a new diet craze every year, and each one promises that if you eat *this* but not *that*, you will quickly drop pounds and lose inches? It's tough to know what to believe. Some people argue that low-carb is the way to go, while others say it's all about eating high-carb. There are fat-free diet plans and diets that encourage you to put butter in your coffee. There's Jenny Craig, Paleo, South Beach, fasting, the cookie diet, the grapefruit diet, Atkins, juicing, the ketogenic diet, the blood type diet, the macrobiotic diet, the Mediterranean diet, raw food, Sugar Busters, Weight Watchers, the Zone, and more. If you've been on any of these diets, you may have initially had some success, but eventually you were probably too hungry, deprived, frustrated, or bored to stay on the plan. I would even argue that dieting makes you fat. (Read on to find out why.)

If you're a serial dieter, you are not alone. There are 108 million dieters in the United States. Every year we spend $21 billion on diet drinks and more than $2 billion on low-calorie foods. The $60 billion diet industry sells books, diet food, diet drinks, and promises that weight loss is within reach. As of early 2017, more than 603 million adults and 107 million children were considered obese, and the numbers are growing (Institute of Health Metrics and Evaluation, 2017). According to the Organization for Economic Co-operation and Development, also known as the OECD (2017), obesity levels are expected to continue to rise, and by 2030 nearly half the population of the United States will be obese.

So if you've tried so many diets—and even had some success—then why do you continue to struggle? In this chapter we'll look at the reasons that diets ultimately don't work in the long term, why willpower has nothing to do with it, the differences between physical and emotional hunger, and the triggers that might be the real reason you are bingeing. I'll also reveal the truth about food addiction. (Hint: it has more to do with your mind than your brain.)

WHY DIETS FAIL

Millions of people are dieting, yet obesity levels keep rising. To understand this, we have to realize that diets fail for biological and psychological reasons. Weight-loss diets are often restrictive. When you take in too few calories, your body becomes more efficient. If your body had a voice, it would say, "What's this? Not enough fuel is coming in. It's time to make the most of these calories. Let's slow our roll." Your metabolic rate decreases, requiring fewer calories to keep your blood flowing, your heart beating, and your organs working. Your body needs fewer calories just for maintenance, so it's much easier to gain weight after you stop dieting. The number on the scale goes up, you try yet another diet, and the cycle continues.

> "In fact, in the long run, dieting often contributes to weight gain."

A significant number of research studies indicate that in the long term, dieting doesn't result in improvements in health, nor does it result in lasting weight loss. In fact, in the long run, dieting often contributes to weight gain. Unbelievable, isn't it? There is plenty of scientific proof that dieting makes you gain weight more easily. In a study of more than two thousand sets of twins, the dieting twin was much more likely to become overweight than the non-dieting twin (Pietiläinen, et al., 2011).

Biology is only part of the reason your diet is failing you. The psychology of eating also creates the overeating and bingeing cycle. When you put those two together, no wonder it's so hard to lose weight and keep it off. The good news is that it's possible to harness the power of your mind to change your body.

Stress and Weight Gain

There's also a correlation between stress and weight gain. The impact of stress on the body has been well documented, so we know there is a connection between stress and the release of a hormone called cortisol, which is linked to weight gain around the stomach. Stress causes the release of cortisol, which makes glucose and then gets stored as belly fat. That's one reason that people under stress are more likely to gain weight.

One study at the Mann Lab, a health and eating lab at the University of Minnesota, followed a group of dieters who consumed the same number of calories on a specific meal plan. Some participants counted calories and others didn't do any calorie counting. Both groups of dieters became more stressed while dieting, whether they were counting calories or not. In other words, simply being on a diet causes stress. Traci Mann, the researcher who conducted this study, notes, "Stress cannot be avoided when you're dieting, because dieting itself causes stress. Dieting causes the stress response that has already been shown to lead to weight gain." If diets cause stress, and stress causes weight gain, then going on a diet may not always be the best way to lose weight.

ARE YOU FEELING STRESSED?

This may seem like a rhetorical question because in today's world most of us encounter many different stressors regularly. But I want you to really think about this. What are the primary stressors in your life? Make a list. Start to notice if when you are feeling those stressors you find yourself bingeing. Awareness is the first step to changing your habits.

Artificial Sweeteners

Another myth about weight loss has to do with artificial sweeteners. Diet soda and other artificially sweetened drinks and foods are marketed as tools for weight loss, yet many studies appear to link them to weight gain instead of weight loss. That's right. Artificial sweeteners can make you gain weight.

"Artificial sweeteners can make you gain weight."

What's really astonishing is that these findings aren't new. Researchers have known of this link between artificial sweeteners and weight gain for decades. The correlation between sugar substitutes and weight gain dates back to the 1970s, when a study of 31,940 nurses revealed that those who used saccharin gained more weight than those who didn't use artificial sweeteners. In the 1980s the American Cancer Society studied 78,694 women and found that the women who used artificial sweeteners gained more weight than those who didn't use them. In that same decade the San Antonio Heart Study concluded that men and women who regularly consumed artificially sweetened drinks had a higher BMI (body mass index) than those who didn't drink those beverages.

All Calories Are Not Created Equal

Another common belief is that all calories are equal. This is the idea that no matter what you eat, whether it's healthy or not, you simply have to expend more calories than you take in. According to this theory, it doesn't matter what you're eating, since a calorie is a calorie is a calorie. Most of us have been taught that to lose 1 pound, you'd have to create a calorie deficit of 3,500 calories. Other studies conclude the same thing—that calories alone are what matters when it comes to weight loss.

Yet our bodies are complex, and not everyone responds the same way. I once treated a woman who insisted that she had to be on a diet and couldn't imagine eating intuitively. She was on Weight Watchers, a plan that asks dieters to count points instead of calories. She used most of her points on processed food such as cookies and protein bars, reasoning that as long as she stayed at her point level, she'd lose weight. She didn't want to give up on the sweets that she loved, and this was a perfect way to eat dessert without guilt. She felt sluggish and tired. Worse, the scale didn't budge.

When she began using her points on fresh whole foods, she started feeling better and lost weight.

This highlights the fact that the quality of the food you're consuming is important to your health and well-being. You can consume 150 calories of ice cream, or you can eat a banana for roughly the same number of calories. Your body gets much more nutrition from the banana than from the ice cream. In 2015 researcher and best-selling author Jonathan Bailor examined more than 1,200 scientific studies to prove that not all calories are equal and revealed conclusively that counting calories isn't an effective tool for weight loss.

So there you have it: Diets don't work.

Artificial sweeteners cause weight gain.

Not all calories are equal.

In fact, most of our commonly held ideas about weight loss are actually myths. When it comes to dieting, the truth is along the lines of what researcher Traci Mann, who runs The Mann Lab, a research laboratory at the University of Minnesota dedicated to studying eating and health habits, concludes: "It is only the rate of weight regain, not the fact of weight regain, that appears open to debate."

IT'S NOT ABOUT WILLPOWER

Weight-loss diets always involve some kind of deprivation, which leads to overeating or bingeing. That's because the anticipation of deprivation, knowing that at some point in the future you're not going to be able to eat your favorite foods, just makes you want them more. This is in line with the results of a study in which dieters had increased cravings for "forbidden foods" while on a diet. One dieter said, "When you're on a diet, it's harder to avoid them [unhealthy foods]. Ice cream is something that I like having once per week, but when I'm on a diet, I want to have it every day."

On the other hand, when people are allowed to eat their forbidden foods, they often eat less. Participants in various studies were asked to eat their forbidden foods as part of their treatment, and the researchers hypothesized that they would not be able to stop. Instead, when told to eat these "addictive" foods, people ate less instead of more—the opposite of what food addiction theory would suggest.

My personal experience with my kids at Halloween is a great example of how this works. My daughter has a friend who isn't allowed to eat sugar. Her mom worries about cavities and overall health and believes that restricting candy is the best way to remain healthy. She thinks sugar is "bad" and doesn't allow it in the house. What do you think that does to her child? I can tell you for sure that it doesn't make the kid think, "Sugar is bad, so I don't want any of that bad stuff." Nope. If anything, she just wants it even more. And that's why, knowing that her Halloween candy was going to be confiscated after trick-or-treating, she began sneaking sugar early in the night. She ate enough candy to wind up with a really bad stomachache. This is a classic example of how the anticipation of deprivation makes you overeat.

Trying to control your intake of candy and other types of food doesn't work. Actually, it usually has the opposite effect, causing you to want more of the forbidden fruit—or candy, in this case. Allowing kids (and yourself) to make their own choices gives them a sense of empowerment and can lead to their making better choices. Sound far-fetched? That very same Halloween night, after a few hours of trick-or-treating, my daughter announced that she was really hungry.

"Have some candy," my husband suggested.

She rolled her eyes. "I don't want candy, Dad. I want *real* food."

I'll admit, that was a proud moment for me. My daughter is a truly intuitive eater, and she recognized what her body needed instead of eating candy. Does it seem utterly impossible that you could ever say something like that? It's not impossible. As Nelson Mandela famously said, "It always seems impossible until it's done."

When you cultivate an intuitive approach to eating, you will naturally be drawn to good, healthy, nutritious food. That's why our daughter wanted "real" food. She was tuned in to what her body wanted, even at the age of ten. My daughter's friend knew her candy was going to be taken away, so she ate too much. My daughter knew she could have as much candy as she wanted, and she didn't want any. This highlights the importance of psychology when it comes to overeating or bingeing.

OVEREATING VERSUS BINGEING

Overeating means "eating to excess" and that's different from binge-ing. There are lots of reasons you may overeat, none of them having to do with feelings. Many Americans overeat on Thanksgiving, which one of my patients cleverly referred to as "National Binge Day." Overeating on that holiday often has to do with food, not feelings, so it's not the same as regular bingeing.

If you don't eat enough and you get to the point where you're ravenous, you may not be able to stop once you start eating and may wind up eating too much. If that's the case, you might think, "Oh, I overdid it, so I'll cut back tomorrow."

> "Unlike overeating, bingeing is being out
> of control with food and usually involves
> remorse, guilt, and shame afterward."

Bingeing, on the other hand, means eating large quantities of food at one time, in a compulsive way, often without enjoying it or even tasting it. Bingeing is a way of coping with something inside. It's about using food for comfort, distraction, or to numb or express pain, anger, anxiety, or anything uncomfortable. Unlike overeating, bingeing is being out of control with food and usually involves remorse, guilt, and shame afterward. You might think, "What's wrong with me?" Not only do you feel bad about what you ate, but you also feel terrible about yourself.

PHYSICAL VERSUS EMOTIONAL HUNGER

I also want to make a distinction between physical and emotional hunger. Here are some signs that you're physically hungry:

- *Growling, gurgling stomach*
- *Feeling light-headed*
- *Getting a headache (especially if you haven't eaten for several hours)*

In contrast, the signs that you're emotionally hungry are located more in your thoughts and your mind than in your body:

- *A specific food "sounds good" or "looks good."*
- *You want to reward yourself.*
- *You want to calm down or feel better.*

Lots of people eat to feel more energized, which isn't emotional hunger, but it's the wrong response to exhaustion. When you're tired, you need to rest. Food won't perk you up for long. Your body needs rest, not food. (And the foods that give you the most energy are actually healthy proteins and vegetables, not sugar-laden snacks that may give you an initial burst of what seems like energy but leave you crashing later.)

THE HIDDEN TRIGGERS

As I mentioned earlier, we are often motivated by what is hidden in our unconscious, meaning it's out of awareness but not out of operation. We have lots of emotions and inner conflicts that we aren't actually aware of, but they have a strong influence over us.

Let me give you an example. Danielle ate perfectly during the day, always healthy choices and salads for lunch. But at night everything went south. Every single night after dinner, she developed what she called a "weakness" for chips. She and her husband were doing a yearlong challenge of not watching TV. Instead they read books. Danielle could never get through her book. She kept getting up and going to the pantry to grab a bag of Doritos. Keep in mind, she ate Doritos only at night and only while she and her husband were reading together. I asked her what she was reading before she started thinking about Doritos.

"Fifty Shades of Grey," she said.

This book triggered all kinds of complicated feelings about intimacy, trust, and sexuality. The book also deals with surrendering control. That really hit home for Danielle—but not when it came to sexuality or intimacy. The idea of submitting control to another person was what got to her.

SURF THE HUNGER WAVE

If you're not sure whether it's emotional or physical hunger, try postponing your meal or snack for three minutes and see what happens. If you're physically hungry, you'll probably get a little bit hungrier, but not so ravenous that you lose control. If you're emotionally hungry, you may become more aware of the underlying emotions that are the driving force behind the urge to eat.

3 min

If that happens, it's time to go surfing. Yes, surfing. No surfboard or ocean required. When that urge to binge or to continue eating strikes—and it can be powerful—imagine that you're surfing the feeling. A wave builds in intensity and becomes more and more powerful, and then it eventually crashes and disappears. Same thing with a binge. It can build up and feel super intense. But it won't stay that intense. It will crest and then diminish in intensity. That's something to keep in mind when you want to eat for emotional reasons. The craving or urge isn't going to last. If you can ride the wave for a little while, it will pass.

When you know whether you're hungry for food or eating to resolve an internal conflict or state, it's easier to make healthy food choices. Three minutes may not sound like a long time, but it can make a big difference. Give it a try.

The truth was that Danielle didn't want to read books for a year. She preferred to "Netflix and chill," but she felt obligated to go along with what her husband wanted. She didn't recognize that reading the book triggered her, because before that uncomfortable feeling of resentment could even reach her awareness, she developed a craving for Doritos.

Danielle finally told her husband how she felt. He had no idea that she wasn't on board with the TV-free lifestyle. He was shocked and surprised that she felt that way, but he was open to compromise. They decided to watch TV together four nights a week one week and three the next week. Danielle got to watch her favorite

Netflix shows and felt more connected to her husband. As for Doritos? She barely ate them. Once she addressed the reason she ate chips, which was as a way of distracting herself from her truth and expressing her annoyance and anger, she stopped craving them. If we'd been focused on chips, nothing would have changed. Those chips were actually a clue to what Danielle was struggling with inside, which we'll explore in the next chapter.

I mentioned earlier that it's impossible to fight an invisible army. As long as what's going on inside remains out of awareness— invisible—you're constantly engaged in a battle that you can't fully understand. Only by recognizing what's truly going on in your head and your heart, by making that army visible, can you battle those destructive ideas, thoughts, and emotions—and win. Danielle's invisible army was the idea that she had to go along with what her husband wanted and not make waves. Yet she also felt a lot of repressed anger toward him for pushing the TV-free zone on her (which was how she saw it). Speaking up helped bring all of this into the open.

Changing your eating habits has nothing to do with willpower and everything to do with identifying your triggers. Michelle, a client in my online program, wrote, "Before Dr. Nina came along, I was beginning to think I was a hopeless case of lazy lack of willpower, and possibly even powerless to food. Now I realize that I'm giving all the 'power' to food to subconsciously avoid the feelings that come along with procrastination due to unrealistic expectations and self-degradation."

For Danielle and Michelle, and countless others, those binges weren't about willpower. Nor were they food addicts. If anything, they had an *eating* addiction, not a *food* addiction. They were addicted to eating as a way of coping, to using food to numb or distract themselves, but they weren't addicted to the actual substance of chips. This is a really important distinction, because there's so much misinformation out there and lots of folks are confused about the concept of food addiction.

So . . . is food addiction real?

THE TRUTH ABOUT FOOD ADDICTION

How many folks do you know who say they're addicted to coffee, alcohol, and cigarettes? They think they're addicted to Instagram, to their phones, to bad relationships, to sex, video games, and gambling. Sometimes it may seem as if the whole world is addicted to something. What's the deal?

The traditional understanding of addiction is that it has to do with the compulsive use of a substance known to the user to be harmful. Usually there's increased tolerance to that substance, meaning that it takes more and more of it to get the same "high." And stopping the use of the substance leads to withdrawal symptoms. The concept of building tolerance applies only to certain drugs that produce physical dependence, but there is no such thing as tolerance to food.

Many who feel powerless over sugar and white flour label themselves as food addicts. They find it especially painful and difficult to grapple with their addiction. After all, alcoholics can stay away from bars and alcohol. Smokers can stay away from cigarettes. Gamblers can stay away from casinos. But no one can give up food. We need to eat to live. And temptation is everywhere—in our homes, gas station mini marts, restaurants, employee lounges, vending machines, the local store, and more.

But is food addiction a real thing?

Some studies make a case for the reward theory of food addiction, which means that certain types of foods are associated with increased dopamine levels. Dopamine is the chemical that mediates pleasure and motivation in our brains. The theory is that sugar and other "hyperpalatable" foods, such as those containing salt and fat, activate the release of dopamine in the brain. People eat something sugary or fatty (or both) and receive a dopamine rush. Food addiction theory points to changes in the brain as evidence of substance addiction.

Sounds reasonable, right? But wait, there's a lot more to the story.

Sugar *does* change our brains. Yet lots of things change our brains. Any activity involving pleasure does so, including sex, exercise, playing sports or video games, and spending time with friends. One study proved that listening to music had the same impact on the brain as cocaine (Salimpoor, 2011). Psychotherapy also changes the brain and can be more effective than medication. Relationships with other people have a direct impact on our brains. In fact, there are many studies that completely refute the notion of food addiction.

What about the studies that show rats prefer sugar to heroin? When given a choice between sugar and heroin, laboratory rats will go for sugar every time. At face value that looks really bad. But think about it: Rats are conditioned to eat for survival. Naturally they'd be attracted to the sugar, which is food, which they need for survival, rather than heroin.

Remember that we have brains, but we also have *minds*. Our brains are the physical control structure of our bodies. They do not operate without the power of our minds, nor do our minds function independently of our brains. Research that focuses exclusively on the brain ignores the powerful influences of our minds, as well as the impact of our culture and society.

"Sugar Is My Personal Crack"

Of course, the science may not matter to someone who *feels* addicted, like Annette, a single mom who was convinced that she was addicted to sugar. As she expressed it, "Sugar is my personal crack." When Annette baked cookies with her young children, she made excuses to get the kids out of the kitchen so she could eat cookie batter in private. She felt like a crazy addict who needed a sugar fix.

Annette was going through a difficult divorce, and she was stuck in an unsatisfying job. Sugary foods provided comfort and distracted her from these problems. She didn't have enough sweetness in her life, so she turned to sugary foods. Her number one source of fun was food.

The more fun we have, the less we need food for that purpose. Annette finalized her divorce, changed jobs, and took up new hobbies. Baking cookies became something fun to do with her kids. Eventually she could taste the batter or just have one cookie without wanting more.

How was it possible for Annette, the self-proclaimed sugar addict, to eat just one cookie? Because it wasn't about the impact of sugar on her brain. When she stopped using food for fun and comfort, she could eat anything in moderation. That had to do with her *mind*.

The feeling of being "addicted" to food is more psychological than physiological. If you have sudden cravings for foods you know are unhealthy, there is always a reason. When you recognize the true triggers, which have nothing to do with the substance of sugar, you can master the addictive behavior.

Danielle ate Doritos to express anger. Her "addiction" was to eating, not to the actual tortilla chips. Annette ate cookies as a source of both pleasure and comfort. For both women, eating was a way of coping with painful or upsetting thoughts and feelings. The first step to reclaiming your power over food is to identify what's going on inside your head and your heart. If you're turning to food, it's not because your brain has formed a physical addiction; it's because your mind is looking for a way to feel better. Even if you automatically eat when you're upset, you can learn to do things differently. When you implement new ways of supporting and soothing yourself, you stop using food to cope.

It takes time, but it's possible—if you put your mind to it.

❀ ❀ ❀

If weight struggles were simply about counting calories or having willpower, then diets wouldn't fail so often. While stress, artificial sweeteners, and empty calories can all contribute to diets not working, the truth is that bingeing often correlates with something going on inside, and food becomes a way to soothe uncomfortable feelings. Emotional hunger tends to spark particular cravings and is often due to hidden triggers that are causing us to use food for comfort. In the next chapter you'll learn which emotions correlate with bingeing on certain foods and how to better identify and express emotions such as anger, sadness, anxiety, and fear.

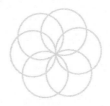

CHAPTER 2

Crack the Code of Emotional Eating

N ow you know that there are hidden emotional triggers that are likely causing your binge eating. But how do you figure out what those triggers are? Well, you may be surprised to hear that certain types of foods often signal particular emotions, and in this chapter I will teach you what I call the Food-Mood Formula. Remember Annette and the cookies? Danielle and the chips? Their cravings were actually clues to their mood. This formula will help you understand if your bingeing stems from a need for comfort or feelings of emptiness—or something else entirely. Are you eating to fill an empty space inside or because you have trouble expressing your anger? We're also going to explore the real meaning behind certain statements such as "I feel fat" or "My clothes are uncomfortable."

Finally, we'll take a good, hard look at the F word. No, not that F word. This one: feelings. Many of us have been taught that our feelings make us weak or that they make other people uncomfortable, so we push them down or ignore them. But feelings are powerful and they want to come to the surface, so when you try to avoid anger, sadness, anxiety, guilt, shame, or loneliness, guess what happens? You turn to food to find relief or comfort from those difficult feelings so that you don't actually have to feel and express them. In this chapter you'll learn healthier ways to express these emotions, because when you give them a voice they become easier to regulate without using food.

THE FOOD-MOOD FORMULA

You probably already know the formula to lose weight: Eat less and exercise more. While that's certainly logical, when it comes to binge eating, it's not about what's logical; it's about what's *psychological*. That's why you have look at what's eating "at" you instead of focusing only on what you're eating.

If you turn to food when you're bored, if you obsess over every calorie, carb, or fat gram, it's always for a reason. By turning to food, you're almost certainly turning away from something else. You may not know what that something else is, but you can figure it out. Even if it feels like you're being triggered by food, something else is going on internally.

This was a difficult concept for Jenna to believe. She was firmly convinced that her problem was all about willpower. She went on her first diet in sixth grade, after a gymnastics coach suggested she drop a few pounds. The very next day she began a diet of grapefruit and hard-boiled eggs, and she quickly lost five pounds. When she returned to normal eating, she gained back those lost pounds. She tried lots of other diets: low-carb, low-fat, Atkins, Weight Watchers, the cookie diet, Master Cleanse, grapefruit, and more. She lost weight every time but regained it when she stopped dieting, adding a few pounds after each diet. This pattern continued through her teenage years and into adulthood.

By the time she came to see me, Jenna was thirty years old and thirty pounds overweight. An attractive woman with glossy chestnut hair and a stylish wardrobe, she felt hopeless about her weight and her life. She never went out on dates, reasoning that if she could not bear to look at herself in the mirror, how could a guy ever find her sexy?

I'll never forget the day Jenna came in for her session and declared, "Maybe some of your other patients are dealing with emotional issues. But I have no willpower. It's about food, not feelings. And I can prove it."

The previous night she had been relaxing and watching TV, when suddenly, as she said, "Ben & Jerry's was calling my name."

She leaned in toward me, speaking emphatically. "Calling My. Name."

She went on to say that nothing was wrong; she wasn't upset or worried about anything, so clearly she was addicted to Chunky Monkey.

"Face it, Dr. Nina," she said, "I'm a food addict and I have no willpower."

I asked Jenna what she was watching on Netflix immediately before she started thinking about ice cream.

"An old rerun of *Charmed*," she answered.

Charmed was her favorite show and she was having a good time, binge-watching episodes. Since she was doing something she enjoyed, there was no reason—or so she thought—that she should have downed a pint of ice cream.

When pressed for details about the episode, she recalled, "It's the show where a demon breaks the bonds between the sisters. He takes away their powers, and they start fighting all the time. It gets really ugly and nasty."

I thought about this, considering Jenna's history. She had difficult relationships with both her sisters. Her older sister rejected all attempts to be close, and her younger sister had no concept of personal space or boundaries. The three of them bickered all the time.

"The show was about sisters who were fighting," I said . . . and waited.

Jenna considered this. She said, "Wow, that's crazy. I didn't even realize that show got me upset about my sisters, but I totally see how it did."

For Jenna, watching the show activated feelings of loss, betrayal, anger, and sadness about her relationship with her sisters. These feelings were so intense that Jenna pushed them out of her mind. Before she was aware that she was upset, she turned to ice cream to cope. Then, by getting angry with herself for eating ice cream, she was taking all the anger and disappointment she felt toward her sisters and directing it toward herself.

Ice cream was not the problem. The problem was Jenna's poor relationship with her sisters. She had a hard time dealing with the painful feelings she had about her siblings. As our work progressed, Jenna learned to identify what she was feeling and thinking instead of reaching for ice cream. She developed new ways of soothing herself and started expressing herself differently. As a result, she stopped bingeing on ice cream.

Today ice cream no longer calls Jenna's name. She isn't obsessed with food, nor is she preoccupied with her size. She maintains a healthy weight and never counts calories or fat grams. She doesn't think about lunch while she's having breakfast or feel bad about herself if she indulges in something she previously considered a "bad" food. In fact, Jenna feels good about herself for the first time in her life. She also started dating and met a really great guy who says of her changing weight, "I loved curvy Jenna and I love thinner Jenna. You're sexy either way."

As she says, "I never thought I could feel this way in my own body. I can't even remember the last time I craved ice cream."

Jenna is living proof that change is possible. Her story also reveals how our deepest emotions can be hidden from us. Those hidden emotions and thoughts have a lot of power over our behavior. In fact, they are often far more powerful than anything we consciously know, think, and believe. Since they are hidden and unconscious, you don't have access to them. But don't worry. I developed a formula to help you figure out exactly what's going on beneath the surface.

Take a moment to think about your last craving. Did you want something smooth like ice cream? Or filling like pizza or cake? Or maybe you grabbed that last bag of chips.

What does it all mean?

In all the years that I've been helping people with eating issues, I started noticing some patterns. No matter what their age, gender, or ethnicity, when it came to cravings, people were drawn to three basic categories of food:

- *Smooth, creamy foods such as ice cream or pudding*
- *Filling foods such as bread, pasta, pizza, cake, or muffins*
- *Crunchy foods such as chips or crackers*

In my work with thousands of men and women, both in my private practice and my online programs, I noticed that when clients said they were craving ice cream, it wasn't really ice cream they wanted—it was *comfort*. So if you want food that is sweet, smooth, and creamy, it's likely that you, too, are in need of nurturing and soothing. This can also apply if you're feeling stressed, because when we feel stressed, we are often in need comfort.

Since ice cream is a clue that you need comfort, the key to change is finding new ways to comfort yourself that don't involve ice cream or sugar. Think about what you'd say to a friend who is sad. I bet you wouldn't tell your friend, "Here, have some ice cream." More likely, you would talk to her or him, showing your interest and support. Later in the book I'll show you how to do this for yourself.

The second category, foods that are filling—such as bread, pasta, pizza, cake, muffins, and burgers—points to loneliness or emptiness, since those types of foods are bulky and fill an inner void. You may feel deprived or lonely, and you eat those foods to symbolically fill up. Boredom is often experienced as loneliness and emptiness, so it may also lead you to eat foods that are filling. If those are the foods you gravitate toward when you're upset, then you need to look at the holes in your life and find new ways to fill them, to fill the emptiness.

Crunchy textures are associated with anger. This category includes chips, pretzels, or basically everything that makes you bite down hard and has a crunch. If chips are your thing, consider what in your life is making you angry, frustrated, or annoyed.

Is it possible to crave all three of these categories at once? Yes. I've had patients who will crave nuts in their ice cream and realize that they are both in need of comfort and feeling angry. That said, there is usually a predominant emotion that needs to be expressed when it comes to bingeing, so you will likely find that you tend to want one of these food categories more often than the others.

Keep in mind that we frequently don't know why we suddenly crave a particular food. What you think of as a "trigger food" actually points to the true trigger: the hidden emotion, need, or conflict. Next time you get a craving, consider whether it's for something smooth, bulky, or crunchy. Chances are, when you identify and respond to the underlying emotion, wish, or need, you'll stop using food to cope.

WHAT IS YOUR TRIGGER EMOTION?

Smooth, creamy foods (ice cream, pudding) = comfort, nurturing, soothing

Filling foods (bread, pasta, pizza, cake) = loneliness, emptiness

Crunchy foods (chips, pretzels, crackers) = anger, frustration

Remember, Jenna didn't know she was upset about her sisters when she heard ice cream calling her name. Danielle was totally unaware of her resentment toward her husband for taking away their TV time, but she took it out on herself by eating Doritos. Consider the possibility that you, too, are redirecting your anger at other people or situations onto yourself.

Shortly after my weekly program on LA Talk Radio first aired, a listener wrote to me, "Dr. Nina, I already know what I'm feeling and I feel my feelings, but nothing ever changes. So clearly *food* is the problem."

If you cry a bucket of tears and you're still sad, there's likely another emotion that's not getting expressed—such as anger. Lots of women convert anger to sadness, because they're taught from an early age that nice girls don't get mad. Many of us only express anger by getting mad at ourselves for what we're eating or what we weigh, when in reality our anger belongs to something or someone else. If you find it easier to feel sad, to cry, and to express yourself with tears, you may be protecting yourself from forbidden feelings of anger.

Or if you're mad, maybe underneath all that anger is a sadness that needs your attention. Men sometimes have a hard time expressing sadness or other vulnerable feelings. They grow up with the message that "boys don't cry," so they tend to turn sadness into anger. Anger is an active emotion, and it can feel better to experience a rush of anger instead of the vulnerability of sadness.

Keep in mind that if you're turning to food to change your mood, you're almost certainly turning *away* from something else. The

Food-Mood Formula only applies to situations when you feel a pull toward food in order to change the way you feel. It's one thing to want chips with your sandwich at lunch; it's a totally different situation when you dive headfirst into a bag of chips and can't stop eating them. There's nothing wrong with having ice cream for dessert. But if you're eating ice cream for comfort, if you find that you can't stop and you feel guilty or ashamed after you eat it, then consider that something psychological is going on.

> "The Food-Mood Formula only applies to situations when you feel a pull toward food in order to change the way you feel."

BODY LANGUAGE

Did you know that your body is talking to you? You just need to be able to hear what it's saying. Take a moment to consider these statements:

- *"I feel fat."*
- *"I ate so much my stomach hurts."*
- *"My clothes are uncomfortable."*
- *"Just thinking about that gives me a headache."*

Each of these sentences has a surface meaning. When we dig a little deeper, we discover some hidden communications. Just as the type of food you habitually turn to can offer a clue as to why you turn to it, so can your words (or language) offer a clue as to what's really going on. So let's start translating!

"I Feel Fat"

Tracy worried that she was doomed to a life of being single. It seemed like all of her friends were either engaged or married. She had a closet full of bridesmaid dresses and no prospects for a second date, much less a husband. She met a lot of guys through a dating app but never felt a genuine spark of attraction or connection. Every week she had a new dating story, each worse than the last.

WHAT ARE YOU TURNING AWAY FROM?

Think about a recent time you found yourself bingeing on a particular food and couldn't stop. Was there anything else going on in your life? Were you angry with someone or something? Were you feeling lonely or in need of comfort? What was your food of choice? Did it correlate with the emotion you were feeling? Next time you find yourself bingeing, take a moment to reflect on what feelings you may be trying to avoid. Below is a list of words to help give you some ideas if you're not sure what exactly you are feeling right now:

Anxiety	**Sadness**	**Anger**	**Disgust**
Concerned	Gloomy	Exasperated	Dislike
Uneasy	Glum	Aggravated	Distaste
Apprehensive	Unhappy	Frustrated	Hatred
Dismayed	Hurt/Hurting	Annoyed	Loathing
Worried	Dejected	Irritated	Revulsion
Alarmed	Grief-stricken	Resentful	Detestation
Distressed	Bereaved	Furious	Nausea
Afraid	Despondent	Incensed	Repugnance
Terrified	Heartbroken	Enraged	
Misgivings	Melancholy	Indignant	
Doubt	Pessimistic	Offended	
Dread	Somber	Outraged	
Horror	Sorry	Cross	
Panic	Blue	Displeased	
Timid	Despairing	Fuming	
Agitated	Downcast	Galled	
Aversion	Forlorn	Huffy	
Consternation	Funk	Maddened	
Foreboding	Morose	Provoked	
Qualms	Morbid	Piqued	
	Troubled	Riled	

Surprise	*Happiness*	*Loneliness*
Amazed	Cheerful	Desolate
Astounded	Content	Empty
Dazzled	Delighted	Abandoned
Awed	Ecstatic	Alone
Bewildered	Elated	Solitary
Disconcerted	Glad	Apart
Overwhelmed	Joyful	Down
Perplexed	Jubilant	Left
Confused	Lively	Rejected
Startled	Overjoyed	Withdrawn
Unsettled	Peaceful	Unsocial
Stunned	Thrilled	
Jarred	Upbeat	
Staggered	Grateful	
Nonplussed	Blissful	
Shaken	Playful	
	Sunny	

One day Tracy told me about her experience with a businessman who'd gone to Harvard, who was smart and funny when they talked on the phone. She agreed to go to a movie with him. When they took their seats at the movie theater, Mr. Harvard noted that the cleaning crew had failed to take the popcorn from the previous screening.

Tracy recalled, "He picked up the container of popcorn and said, 'Look, free popcorn,' and then he started eating it." She made a face of disgust, aghast at the memory. "That was just the beginning of the night. Trust me, it went downhill from there."

Tracy feared that she was never going to find anyone. She worried about ending up in an apartment alone, with only her dog for company. She added, "I feel so fat today."

Fat is a substance, not a feeling. If you feel fat, that's usually code for something else. In Tracy's case she was feeling hopeless, disappointed, and lonely. Feeling "fat" is different for everyone and changes according to the situation. Maybe you're afraid that the intensity of your emotions, needs, or wants is too much and too big for others. "I feel fat" can also be code for something like, "I'm afraid I want, need, and/or feel too much." Or it could be that you feel guilty for taking up space in the world and/or having appropriate needs and demands.

Ask yourself what you might be avoiding. What emotions are you pushing away? What feels like too much or what is overwhelming you? When you translate the expression of "feeling fat" into fears, worries, anxieties, and other states of mind, you can deal with them so they go away for good. I'll show you exactly how to do that later in the book.

"I Ate So Much My Stomach Hurts"

The night that Linda broke up with her long-term girlfriend, she ordered a large pizza because that's all she could think about in her state of despair. Over the course of the next few hours, she ate the entire pizza by herself.

"I ate so much it hurt," she said. "I was in so much pain I literally couldn't move. It was horrible."

Linda was focused on her painfully full stomach, which took her away from the heartache about the breakup. By eating until she was in physical pain, she converted emotional hurt to physical hurt. By filling up until she was stuffed, she symbolically filled the void she felt from the loss of her girlfriend.

If you ever feel so full it hurts, ask yourself what is hurting your feelings. Healing your heart is the key to having a peaceful relationship with food. Only after Linda grieved the end of her relationship did she stop bingeing.

Loneliness can be experienced as emptiness. If you're using food to fill an internal void or if you eat until it hurts, you may be turning the ache of loneliness into an actual physical pain. Physical pain is easier to manage and get rid of than emotional pain. We see this all the time in kids. Children don't typically say, "I don't want to go to school because I didn't finish my homework and I'm afraid of getting in trouble." Instead they say they have a stomachache.

When one of my daughters complained that her tummy was hurting, I ruled out the usual suspects: food poisoning, the flu, or allergies. It turned out she was nervous about starting classes at a new dance academy. She worried about fitting in and being good enough. She didn't tell me about this worry in words. Instead, her anxiety expressed itself as a painful tummy.

I knew for sure that there was nothing physically wrong because talking through her anxieties stopped the pain. When she felt better emotionally, her stomach also felt better. The same thing will happen for you when you start recognizing and processing your hidden or painful truths. It's all about honoring your truth, even if it's painful. Once you do that, you stop coping with food, distracting with food, numbing with food, and more. That's when you're finally free from the prison of dieting.

"My Clothes Are Uncomfortable"

Sylvie often mentioned how uncomfortable she felt in her clothes. At home she wore leggings and oversize shirts, which felt relaxed and comfortable. Her work clothes felt too tight and restrictive. Sylvie didn't want to buy new clothes that fit better. She desperately wanted to lose weight. She often began her sessions by talking about how tight her clothes were and how uncomfortable she felt in them. She complained, "I hate how my clothes fit. My pants feel so tight and uncomfortable."

I wondered if she was talking about something other than clothes when she talked about being uncomfortable. What about her life was causing her to feel uncomfortable and constricted? What in her world wasn't a good fit?

Sylvie looked skeptical. "Dr. Nina," she said, "not everything has to have a deeper meaning. Sometimes tight clothes are just tight clothes."

I acknowledged that she certainly had a point. Even Freud supposedly said that sometimes a cigar is just a cigar (and not always a phallic object). I asked her to humor me and think a little bit about where in her life she might feel trapped and uncomfortable. Since she didn't have this problem at home, maybe there was something about her work situation that was causing some discomfort.

"I can't do anything about my career," she said. Sophie was a physician with a full practice and a hectic schedule. "I've invested ten years and a ton of money into my job, and I can't just walk away."

Sylvie grew up knowing she was going to become a physician. Both her parents were doctors, as were her brothers. She preferred to study art history but didn't want to disappoint her parents.

After medical school she joined a demanding Beverly Hills medical practice that was not a good "fit" for her personality. Sylvie talked about the tightness of her clothing as a way of expressing that her job wasn't a good fit.

As we explored how uncomfortable Sylvie felt in her career, she felt an enormous sense of relief. "It's like a tight belt was loosening up," she exclaimed.

She enrolled in an art history class at a local community college and had something she looked forward to doing. Eventually she left the Beverly Hills medical group and opened up her own practice. She stopped eating for comfort and lost weight without much effort. For the first time in her life, Sylvie was able to keep the weight off without dieting or willpower.

I find that when we explore the symbolism of what's going on with food, we always discover other meanings. Feeling "uncomfortable" can refer to a range of different feelings and may actually mean anxious, awkward, uneasy, tense, worried, edgy, restless, embarrassed, and more. When you're curious about what is making you physically uncomfortable, you're more likely to figure out what's feeling emotionally uncomfortable. Then you can focus on the root problem and work to make changes.

"Thinking About That Gives Me a Headache"

A year after his divorce was final, Adam started to think about meeting someone new. He had met his ex-wife in college twenty years ago. The world had drastically changed since the last time he was single.

"There were no cell phones the last time I wanted to ask someone out," Adam said. "Now I'm supposed to find a girlfriend by swiping right, or left, or whatever. Just thinking about it gives me a headache."

If you have a headache, you pop a Tylenol or an Advil and the pain fades eventually. Painful thoughts are another matter entirely. Adam's headache didn't go away when he took medication. His headache meant that the idea of dating was painful. What were the rules? What if he met someone who didn't like his kids? What if someone wanted more kids? What if he got his heart broken again? These thoughts gave him a headache, a stomachache, and sometimes made him break out in a sweat.

Every Saturday night Adam holed up in his condo and spent the night eating pizza and drinking beer. As we processed his dating anxieties, he started going out. Eventually he met new people and began having fun instead of scarfing down pizza. Once that happened, he lost weight and stopped getting headaches. Although Adam has not yet found the right woman, he's now confident that she's out there.

There are so many ways that our bodies express or protect us from painful or difficult feelings. When you identify and process what is weighing on you, the weight will come off more easily than you ever imagined.

WHAT DOES YOUR BODY LANGUAGE REALLY MEAN?

"I feel fat." = *Maybe your feelings are "too much" or you feel like you are taking up "too much" space.*

"I ate so much my stomach hurts." = *Maybe you are trying to fill an internal void or you are feeling anxious.*

"My pants are tight and uncomfortable." = *Maybe you are feeling trapped and uncomfortable in your job or elsewhere in your life.*

"Just thinking about it gives me a headache." = *Maybe there is something too painful to address in your life.*

THE "F" WORD

Let's talk about the "F" word. Don't worry, this isn't about to get R-rated. I'm actually talking about another "F" word: feelings.

Do you ever get the idea that you're supposed to avoid feelings? That feelings are bad? Weak? Most of us believe that we should kick those pesky feelings to the curb. We're told we're weak if we experience our feelings and strong if we push them away. The basic message is: *There's something wrong with feelings.*

Angry? You must have an anger management problem.

Sad? You're depressed, so take an antidepressant.

Anxious?	There's a pill for that too.
Scared?	Be strong! Fight! Don't give in to fear!
Happy?	Maybe you're a little too happy. Hypomanic, maybe? Bipolar?

No wonder so many of us have a hard time recognizing that emotions, needs, desires, and reactions are part of being human. A feeling is simply a reaction to a situation. It's a response, not a character flaw. With all the cultural prohibitions against feelings, it's no surprise that so many of us have difficulty identifying and processing our emotions. What are the feelings we want to avoid? In no particular order they include: anger, sadness, anxiety, guilt, shame, loneliness, and one other, which I'll get to later. (I think it's going to surprise you.)

Anger

Beth had a love-hate relationship with the scale for much of her adult life. She married her college boyfriend, Bryan, while he was in medical school. Bryan built a successful plastic surgery practice, and Beth stayed at home to raise three daughters. Her weight was stable throughout the years she was bringing up her girls. She loved being a stay-at-home mom, and she didn't worry too much about her weight. She'd recently become an empty nester, and that happiness now seemed like a lifetime ago. Beth was preoccupied with losing the twenty pounds she had gained over the past year, when her last child went off to college.

"I have so much to be happy about," she told me. "I'm truly blessed. Bryan and I are in great shape financially. Our kids are all healthy and happy. So what's my problem? Why can't I stop eating?"

Beth ate "perfectly" all day: a bowl of bran cereal with nonfat milk for breakfast, carrots or string cheese at midday, a salad at lunch, and a healthy dinner of either fish or chicken and vegetables. It was only at night, after dinner, that she found herself wandering into the kitchen, looking for something to eat, and soon losing control.

"I'm so good all day," she said. "Why do I mess it all up at night? I'm not even hungry."

She usually ate potato chips or popcorn at night. Beth cringed as she admitted that she often consumed an entire family-size bag of chips in one sitting.

She tried to find a physical reason for her cravings. "I wonder if I just have a thing for salt? I never go for anything sweet. You could put a bowl of ice cream in front of me and I wouldn't be tempted in the least."

I told Beth that her food choices might give us a clue about what was going on with her emotionally. If you recall the Food-Mood Formula, you probably already figured out that Beth's preference for crunchy foods like chips, popcorn, or pretzels often is associated with some kind of anger. She was definitely pissed off about something.

Beth wasn't on board with this idea. "You're saying that if I eat something crunchy that means I'm angry. But I don't feel angry. Except I'm kind of mad at myself for losing control at night. Besides, I'm not an angry person."

I told Beth that being angry didn't make her an angry person. It made her a person who was angry. Beth looked doubtful.

By our next session, Beth had clearly continued to give this more thought. "Last night Bryan texted that he was running late, even later than usual. I understand he's busy, with a lot of demands on his time. It's always been that way, since he was in med school. But right after I heard from him, I went to the kitchen for chips."

"Sounds like you had some feelings about his lateness."

Beth sighed. "I shouldn't have feelings about it. That's part of the deal, being a doctor's wife. Even when the girls were little, he was never home before seven or eight o'clock at night. Besides, I can't do anything about it."

I said, "You seem to think that just because you know something logically, you shouldn't have any feelings about it."

"Shouldn't I be able to make myself feel differently about things, if I know there's nothing I can do?"

I explained that logic doesn't change emotions. You cannot talk yourself out of, or into, feelings. It's impossible to tell yourself not to feel upset and then immediately feel different. Beth struggled with this concept. She had always felt like a failure for not doing or feeling what she "knew" was best for her. I was offering a radically new perspective.

Every time Beth crunched down on some chips, she was expressing her anger. Later she took that anger out on herself for having no willpower. She denied her anger and then turned it against herself. She had spent years denying her true feelings, then attacking herself for her weight or for eating the wrong thing.

Beth slowly got in touch with her feelings toward her husband. She admitted to herself that she had always resented how Bryan made work more of a priority than family. During those years of raising the girls, she was busy taking them to dance classes, art lessons, equestrian lessons, and more. She never noticed how much Bryan was gone. Now that the girls were grown, she was alone in an empty house and more than a little resentful. Food distracted her from those upset feelings.

Underneath Beth's problem with food was a problem in her marriage. She didn't feel like a priority to her husband. Once she became interested in what she was feeling, instead of what she was eating, she set her sights on creating change. She made an appointment with a marriage therapist and started dealing with those marital issues. It didn't take long before she stopped eating chips.

Let me ask you something: *What if I took away your ability to be mad at yourself for the number on the scale, or for polishing off that plate of nachos?* Who would you be mad at? Imagine what would happen if you couldn't direct that resentment, anger, or frustration at yourself.

Once you know that, you've got to own it. That doesn't mean confronting anyone. If you're upset with your boss, it's probably not a good career move to speak out. There are times when you may actually confront a person, but often the most important thing is to acknowledge your feelings to yourself, for yourself, and express yourself in a healthy way.

HOW TO EXPRESS ANGER

You can't stuff down your feelings with food. Nachos, cookies, or bags of chips won't get rid of your anger. You can't ignore your feelings, drop them, positive-think them away, let them go, or deny them. As counterintuitive as it may seem, there's only one way to get rid of feelings: to feel them.

Identifying a feeling is different from actually expressing it. Identifying an emotion sounds neutral, as if you're stating a fact. For example, if you say "I'm really upset" in the same basic way you might say "It's really warm today," then you're probably identifying your anger but not feeling it. That's thinking your anger instead of feeling it.

Feeling emotion is different. It requires intensity and conviction. That means having a heart-pounding, adrenaline-pumping physical sensation. Think, heat.

"I am really upset!"

That's ultimately what stops those feelings. We see this all the time in young children, who may cry out of disappointment or have a tantrum, but when they're done, it's over. The storm has passed and it's on to the next activity.

I'm not suggesting that you wail and cry, beating your fists on the floor like a toddler. Acknowledging, validating, and expressing yourself isn't being childish. It's honoring your truth. So phone a friend. Write in a journal. Take a kickboxing class. Get those feelings out instead of turning them on yourself. Your anger (and all your other feelings) needs your attention, not your condemnation.

Sadness

Maryam was living her dream life. She spent years climbing the corporate ladder and was president of a large corporation. Her husband Daniel took care of their twin girls and was a source of support. In her professional capacity Maryam commanded the respect of people all over the world. In her private life she wasn't close to many people.

Her parents were retired and lived in the San Francisco area but rarely visited Los Angeles, where Maryam lived. They traveled all over the world for pleasure, often for weeks at a time, yet it was "too difficult" to fly down to Los Angeles. As a result, they had not visited for three years and only saw her via Skype. In contrast, they spent a lot of time with their other grandchildren, two boys who were the sons of Maryam's estranged brother. When she was growing up, her parents had clearly favored her brother. Their gender preference for boys now extended to their grandchildren.

Maryam recalled that whenever she wept or reacted with sadness as a child, her father would reach for his belt. "I'll give you something to cry about!" he'd say. She quickly learned to stifle her tears. She also internalized her father's anger toward anything painful and sad.

"Can you believe my parents?!" fumed Maryam. "They don't care about my kids at all. How can they do this to their grandkids?"

I privately shared her disbelief and anger. Their lack of interest was utterly incomprehensible. "Not just their grandkids," I observed.

Maryam made a dismissive motion with her hand. "I'm an adult," she said. "I can handle it, but it really bothers my kids. They think my parents don't like them."

We sat and reflected in a moment of shared sadness. Maryam broke the silence, saying, "I don't know how I got off on that tangent about my parents. They're never going to change, so there's no point in even talking about them. What's really on my mind is that I can't stop eating chocolate. I'm completely out of control."

I explained to Maryam that the point of expressing feelings isn't to change the situation. We express feelings to change the way we feel about the situation. When someone we love passes away, we don't say, "There's no point in grieving since it's not going to bring him or her back to life." We mourn and go through the stages of grief so that we will feel better about our loss.

Maryam nodded. "I see your point. Except that I'm not sad. I'm not mourning a loss. I'm mad at my parents for being such crappy parents and grandparents. And I'm mad at myself for eating chocolate."

Several months later, Maryam was diagnosed with an autoimmune disease that was painful and potentially life-threatening. I worried about her and was also struck by her stoicism as she told me the diagnosis. She was lucky, she assured me, that she was diagnosed early and was able to manage her symptoms with medication. Maryam continued to work at her demanding job during this difficult time. Her husband was a constant source of support and love.

"He's all I need," she told me. "He's the only person I can count on to be there for me. I don't need anyone else."

In the following weeks, Maryam started to look exhausted. One day she sat on the couch and looked at me, her eyes filling with tears. "I'm going through the worst, scariest time in my life," she said, "and only two of my friends have bothered to text and see how I'm doing."

My heart went out to Maryam, whose bravado and tough attitude were beginning to crack. She stared at her hands, examining her manicured nails for a long moment. "What's wrong with me?" she asked. "Why don't people care about me? My own parents don't even care to visit me, and you know what they're doing right now? They're in Europe on a river cruise."

Tears ran down her cheeks. She was finally getting in touch with the pain of rejection from her parents. For years, Maryam buried these feelings and ate chocolate for solace. She was finally grieving the sadness of a lifetime of rejection.

At our next session Maryam shared that she had ordered chocolate soufflé at a recent business dinner. "Then I realized I didn't want it," she said. "I want something I can never have. I want parents who actually give a damn about me."

Maryam was finally in touch with her sadness. She became kinder to herself and began comforting herself with words instead of chocolate (although she allowed herself the occasional piece of See's candy). It didn't take long for her to lose weight.

"I'm a Dude. I Don't Have Feelings."

Men grow up with the message that emotions such as anger are acceptable. In contrast, vulnerable emotions such as sadness, loneliness, or fear aren't okay. In fact, the very existence of those emotions is perceived as feminine or weak.

One of my male patients once said, "I'm a dude. I don't have feelings."

I said, "Well, dude, yeah, you do. Because human beings have feelings, and you're human. And those feelings need your attention."

John Bukenas, host of a podcast called *Let's Reverse Obesity*, once told me, "It is a struggle with emotions. Men aren't allowed to show certain emotions that could be perceived as feminine."

That was certainly the case with Tom, who worked all his life at a printing company. He passed up time with his family so that he could get his work accomplished. Tom expected his loyalty to be appreciated and rewarded, but when the company underwent reorganization, he lost his job. Tears filled his eyes as he told me about the injustice he felt at this turn of events, and how insignificant he appeared to be, despite all his years of service and hard work. He told me they were "angry tears" and that he wasn't sad.

The way to get rid of sadness is to feel it, to cry, sometimes with tears running silently down your cheeks, and sometimes with the shoulder-shaking sobs that rack your body. Whether you are a man or a woman, it's important to allow yourself to feel sadness and to release it. Mark Twain was once asked, during a particularly brutal winter, if he thought the rain would ever stop. "It always does," he said.

And like the rain, pain also comes to an end. It always does.

Anxiety

Anxiety refers to a range of emotions including fear, worry, and phobias. Many of us are beset with anxiety. We get scared of being fired from our jobs. We worry about being rejected. We think about the worst-case scenarios. We have irrational fears about being in public or about flying. These worries mask deeper anxieties, such as powerlessness and vulnerability.

Fear of getting fat, for example, is not just about food. That anxiety expresses fear of being powerless and helpless in life. Fear of flying is a fear of what happens if you don't have total control. If you're in a situation you can't control, it may be easier to focus on your powerlessness over food rather than over the situation.

Ellyn, a college student, needed to straighten her hair before a party, but her flat iron had broken. She lived in a college dorm and decided that she was going to ask her roommate, Jane, if she could borrow her flat iron. Then she worried, "What if Jane doesn't want to lend it to me?"

That thought led to more fears. "What if I borrow her flat iron and it breaks? What if she gets mad at me and we have a big fight? What if everyone in the dorm takes her side? What if they all hate me? What if I never make any new friends?"

At that moment Jane walked in the room. Ellyn burst out, "You know what, Jane? You can just keep your stupid flat iron!"

Jane blinked in confusion, bewildered.

Ellyn never went to the party. Instead she stayed in her dorm room and ate a giant bowl of pasta.

This shows how people can have very real feelings about something that has not happened and may not actually happen. Anxiety is an emotion characterized by worrying about some future situation and that often causes physical symptoms such as a rapid heartbeat, sweating, shaking, or dizziness. Why is anxiety a trigger? Anxiety feels uncomfortable, and since food has a sedative effect, you may eat to relax and calm down. This is especially likely to be true if you often find yourself bingeing on carbohydrates such as bread, pasta, or anything that can make your body drowsier or more relaxed. Instead of eating to relax, soothe your body by exercising, stretching, doing guided meditation, or soaking in a bath or hot tub. When your body is relaxed, your mind will follow. A relaxed body and mind allow for deeper investigation into the roots of your anxiety or conflicts. Calming your body through meditation or other means is valuable and necessary for relaxation, and a relaxed and open mind is essential to stop future anxiety.

"What If" Versus "What Is"

Most anxiety has a "what if" component. **"What if"** is about **fear** and has to do with believing that punishment, rejection, or deprivation lies ahead. For example:

What if I gain five pounds after eating that cookie sandwich/pizza/cake?

What if I go out with that guy and he turns out to be a complete jerk?

What if I ask someone out on a date and she rejects me?

What if I ask my boss for a raise and she gets mad?

What if I make a mistake and get fired?

What if I say the wrong thing?

When you have here-and-now emotions about future events that may or may not actually happen, you're more likely to eat for distraction or comfort. Fear intensifies anxiety and leads to overeating or bingeing, which causes you to replace anxiety about a future event with anxiety about weight, calories, and so forth.

In contrast, **"what is"** is about **reality**. It references what is known and validated. When you're grounded in what is actually happening, you're less likely to feel anxious, worried, or upset. And when you feel good, you don't use food to cope.

Challenge anxiety by remembering what you know to be true about the situation and about yourself. Think about how you have handled difficult situations in the past. Remembering your strengths and capabilities diminishes fear because when you recall the tough times you have already been through, and you know that you can survive and thrive after adversity, you feel stronger and less scared about the future.

I know this to be true from personal experience. A few years ago I was diagnosed with early-stage breast cancer. Luckily, I didn't have to endure the invasive and horrible treatment that so many women have to undergo, and I had a lumpectomy and radiation. When the treatment was behind me, I wanted some kind of visual reminder that I had survived this adversity. I decided to get a tattoo of roses, complete with thorns, as a reminder that even though there are moments and situations that are thorny, times that hurt you and cause pain, there is also beauty. Roses, after all, are bigger and more beautiful than their thorns.

Whenever I encounter a challenging, painful situation, I think of my tattoo and feel a surge of confidence, remembering that I have faced tremendous challenges in my life and have overcome them, and I will overcome this as well. Think about what that kind of reminder may be for you—some talisman or symbol that reminds you that you are a warrior and a survivor, even if you don't feel like one (you're here, aren't you?)—and you can get through whatever challenges you're facing. That may be a ring, a bracelet, a tattoo, or anything that reminds you of your strength and abilities.

Loneliness

Roberta had an active social life but felt something was missing. She enjoyed attending art gallery openings, movies, and the theater with her friends. Yet she always sensed that people were simply tolerating her presence instead of enjoying her company. Social interactions were exhausting, so the first thing she did when she arrived home was to head straight for the pantry.

Roberta felt a profound loneliness even when she was with other people. The state of loneliness means wanting to connect with others. Being in the same room as other people isn't the same as feeling safe and fulfilled. If you experience profound emptiness and disconnection, then food is an easy way to symbolically fill up. It's definitely a solution, but not a good one.

The solution is shifting from loneliness to solitude. Solitude is about being alone with a nurturing, loving, supportive part of yourself, an inner voice that's always available to offer understanding and reassurance.

> "If you eat when you're bored, maybe you're actually lonely."

Loneliness is sometimes mistaken for boredom. One of the comments I hear most often is something along the lines of, "I wasn't feeling anything emotional. I was just bored." If you eat when you're bored, maybe you're actually lonely. The key to stopping boredom in its tracks is to be active and productive. Eating is something to do, but it doesn't solve the real problem. When you meet the true need, whether it's loneliness or boredom, you stop using food for comfort or distraction.

Guilt

My friend Amanda and I met for a Krav Maga class recently. Krav Maga is an Israeli form of martial arts that focuses on self-defense and street fighting. Needless to say, it's extremely challenging.

"Great class," I said as we walked to our cars.

"It was," agreed Amanda. "But I feel so guilty for leaving Jonathan with the kids. Here I am at Krav having fun and he's at home giving the twins a bath."

Amanda felt guilty about doing something for herself while her husband was home with the kids. Guilt can be about something that you did or didn't do. Guilt also references behavior and actions. You feel guilty when you think you've done something wrong, or when you choose not to take action. Guilt sounds like, "I've done something really bad and wrong," or "I should have done something different."

Depletion Guilt

There are different types of guilt. Amanda was experiencing what's called **depletion guilt**. This involves a sense that if you do something for yourself or meet your own needs, you're taking something away from others, depleting them in some way. In Amanda's case, by going to Krav Maga, she felt as if she was burdening her husband with childcare duties. (The way I see it, that's called fatherhood, but Amanda's relationship is a whole other story.) Some other examples of depletion guilt include:

- *If I leave my husband, he'll be miserable. I can't do that to him.*
- *I'm turning down that great job in Chicago. My mom was so upset when my sister moved to New York. I can't do that to her. I'll stay in L.A. even if it's not the right thing for me.*
- *I want to be an artist, but my parents will be so disappointed if I don't go to law school. They've been counting on me to join the family law firm since I was born.*

Self-Guilt

Another type of guilt is called **self-guilt**, which is the guilt you feel as a result of actually being or existing in the world, for having any needs. The sense is that by needing anything—food, nurturing, comfort, security, and love—you're exposing a deficiency in yourself and even a belief that it's fundamentally wrong to have needs. Self-guilt sounds like:

- *I shouldn't be so hungry/tired.*
- *I'll go to whatever movie/restaurant/vacation you prefer. It makes no difference to me where we go.*
- *Sure, I'll babysit for you tomorrow night. It's not a problem to cancel my plans.*

This often involves a sense that your needs/wants will be burdensome to others. You go out of your way to put the needs of others before your own. All of these types of guilt are related to food issues because of the mechanism of displacement. Instead of feeling guilty about something in our lives, we feel guilty for what we're eating. And binge eating is a way of comforting or distracting from the guilt.

Shame

Guilt is different from shame, which is about who you are as a person. Shame has to do with your essential character. Whereas guilt sounds like, "There's something wrong with what *I did*," shame sounds like, "There's something really bad and wrong with *me*."

"I was really bad last night. I ate pizza *and* cookies." If you feel guilty and/or ashamed for eating, what crimes are you accusing yourself of?

If you feel "good" when you eat healthy food and "bad" when you eat something you think you shouldn't have eaten, then your sense of self is overly tied to food. If you feel shame for eating pizza, ice cream, or whatever, stop and ask yourself, "why did I eat it?" What was going on? And, by the way, there isn't anything inherently wrong with eating junk foods. If you eat something decadent every so often and you enjoy it, that's great. Life is meant to be lived and enjoyed, and that includes sometimes eating yummy foods that aren't always super healthy or nutritious.

If you overeat or binge on a regular basis, whether it's on healthy foods or unhealthy foods, and you're eating as a way of managing deeper intolerable feelings, then it's important to know what's leading you toward food rather than focusing on what you're eating. Eating as a way of managing emotions is a temporary solution to the problem. It's not "the" problem.

Eating unhealthy food has come to be associated with "being bad," and eating healthy food has come to mean that you're "being good." Thought of in this way, what you eat is connected to your character. When you take a step back and think about that, it seems a bit ludicrous that your goodness or worthiness is tied to what you choose to put in your mouth. Yet we say things all the time that indicate that we see eating as practically a criminal act:

- *I was so bad last night. I ate pizza.*
- *I'm hungry for fried chicken, but I've been so good today. I don't want to ruin it.*
- *I can't eat in front of my friends. They'll think I'm a pig.*

How you relate to your emotions, needs, wants, and thoughts reveals a lot about your relationship with different aspects of yourself. There are three basic parts: the self, the prosecutor, and the defense attorney.

The **self** refers to the part of you that has needs, wants, wishes, emotions, and conflicts. When you say, "I was feeling mad/sad/glad/afraid," that's your "self" talking. It's usually the part that is vulnerable to judgment and criticism.

The **prosecutor** is relentlessly critical, finding fault with your thoughts, feelings, wishes, and needs. When you refer to yourself in the second person (calling yourself "you"), it's usually the critic talking.

The **defense attorney** is the part that can be calm, understanding, and supportive. Often that's the part that can show up for other people but not for you. I find that a lot of my patients are available to their friends and family in a warm, open way but are unable to be as accepting of themselves as they are of others.

Ideally, when you experience a need, wish, emotion, or conflict, you respond with comforting or soothing words. All too often, things aren't ideal. When you don't know how to soothe yourself, you're more likely to turn to food for comfort. That in turn leads to judgment ("How could you have eaten that?" or "You failed!") and the cycle continues. Responding to yourself in a soothing way is the key.

BINGEING IS NOT A CRIMINAL ACT

Are you eating as a way of escaping a loud inner voice? Do you tell yourself things like:

- *You're not good enough.*
- *You don't deserve to be happy.*
- *You're such a loser.*

Food can momentarily take you away from that internal critic, the part that attacks your spirit and stops you from living your best life. (Hint: A quick way of identifying your inner critic is to catch when you talk to yourself in the second person. For example, when you say things like, "You're a loser" rather than "I'm a loser.")

Here's how to silence that mean voice:

Imagine a mental courtroom. You're well acquainted with your internal prosecutor/critic. Now cultivate an internal defense attorney. When the prosecutor says you're not good enough, OBJECT. Then take the floor and demand evidence for these accusations. Remember, a judge will tell you:

Feelings are not facts.

Feelings are not admissible as evidence. If you feel like there's something wrong with you, challenge that notion. If you feel like you should be in a different place in your life, challenge that too. Give your defense attorney an equal opportunity to be heard. When the internal prosecutor accuses you of not being good enough, don't accept it as the truth. Demand that the prosecutor define "good enough." (By the way, that is subjective and NOT a number on the scale.) What criteria form the basis of this accusation? Is it your weight? What else?

Present alternative evidence to the court.

Think about how you actually live your life. If you're reading this, there is likely a part of you that is proactive, hopeful, and willing to consider new perspectives. If you have tried and failed at many diets, you're not a failure—you're really tenacious. When you weigh the evidence and judge for yourself, chances are you'll come to a different conclusion from the one you'd reach if you only looked at yourself through the eyes of a prosecutor.

Stop punishing yourself for crimes you haven't committed.

Liberate yourself from that inner prosecutor and feel better about yourself, so you won't use food for comfort or distraction or restrict food to give yourself a sense of well-being.

Vulnerability/Helplessness

Helplessness is a feeling that most people cannot bear to experience, either on its own or because it intensifies other painful or upsetting feelings. Being helpless is defined as: 1) unable to help oneself; 2) weak or dependent; 3) deprived of strength or power; 4) incapacitated. The state of helplessness is connected to vulnerability and dependency, both of which can be extremely uncomfortable.

Corinne's insurance company made it difficult for her to have access to her benefits. As a result, she couldn't see the therapist of her choice unless she paid out of pocket. Her appeals to the insurance company were unsuccessful and she felt powerless. Corinne began to restrict food, which was a way of expressing her deprivation over not being able to see the therapist she wanted to see—and also a way of coping with the helplessness she felt because she was taking an action. Inevitably she would completely lose control and binge on pretzels, turning her helplessness about the insurance situation into helplessness over food.

Addiction specialist Lance Dodes, a psychoanalyst and author who writes extensively on addiction, says that people with addictions are often overwhelmed by helpless feelings and driven to the addictive behavior as a way of reversing that helplessness. As he explains, "Addiction has long been deeply misunderstood in both our culture and clinical practice. Rather than being a reflection of impulsivity or self-destructiveness, or a result of genetic or physical factors, addiction can be shown to be a psychological mechanism that is a subset of psychological compulsions in general." He notes that addictive urges are never random, and when one understands the emotional factors that produce them, addiction can be mastered.

Dodes proposes that the feeling of helplessness is the foundation of most painful and upsetting emotions. When you're doing something like eating, you're taking an action and thus diminishing that sense of powerlessness. Similarly, psychoanalysts Axel Hoffer and Dan Buie believe that helplessness "underlies other intolerable feelings such as incompetence, shame, embarrassment, humiliation, weakness, panic, isolation, rage and hate." Thought of in this way, helplessness itself is a traumatic condition. Anger, productivity, withdrawal, and denial are ways of distracting from helplessness:

- *Anger: Anger is an active emotion, whereas helplessness is a passive emotion. You may get angry with yourself for your weight or be upset with yourself for what you're eating or the amount, as a way of avoiding your sense of helplessness.*

- *Productivity: Being busy is another way of turning passive to active. Focusing on achievements, productivity, and being a slave driver to yourself are all strategies to distract from helplessness. Thinking about food, weight, and calories are examples of focusing on "doing" rather than "feeling."*

- **Withdrawal:** *Withdrawal is a way of denying helplessness. Avoiding people and staying in the house, isolating and eating take-out food, is one form of withdrawal.*

- **Denial:** *If you tell yourself that what makes you feel helpless "isn't a big deal," you may be denying your true feelings in order to minimize the reality of the situation. This is a way of dismissing your feelings. It's easier to focus on something you can control, such as your weight, than it is to feel a profound sense of helplessness.*

The good news is that when you're curious about yourself instead of critical, you're more likely to figure out what you're feeling. Recall a time you felt helpless when you were a child. Maybe you couldn't stop your parents from getting a divorce or there was a time when you weren't treated fairly or felt you weren't heard. How did that situation or moment make you feel? That same experience of helplessness gets revived when something in your present activates those feelings from the past. Are you feeling those same feelings you did when you were young? If so, you are likely feeling the emotion of helplessness or vulnerability. When you recognize your feelings, you can respond to yourself with comfort words instead of with comfort food.

SPEAK YOUR MIND

Once you identify your feelings, it's time to start expressing them. When you keep your feelings bottled up, any expression of emotions feels like way too much. Everything feels too intense and impossible to tolerate. Big feelings lead to binges. The more adept you become at recognizing your emotions and gauging their intensity, the easier it is to regulate them. When you're able to identify what you're feeling, notice the intensity of what you're feeling, and express your emotions verbally, you're not going to stuff them down with food.

The following are all variations of anger, sadness, anxiety, guilt, shame, loneliness, and helplessness, from relatively innocuous to powerful. (Note that some emotions have more variations than others.) This helps you to identify and gauge the intensity of your emotions. Speaking your feelings makes it less likely that you'll turn them on yourself.

Give Anger a Voice

I'm exasperated (because/when/that) . . .

(e.g., "I'm exasperated when I ask people to clean up after themselves and they don't do it.")

I'm aggravated . . .

I'm frustrated . . .

I'm annoyed . . .

I'm irritated . . .

I resent . . .

I'm angry . . .

I'm furious . . .

I'm incensed . . .

I'm enraged . . .

Give Sadness a Voice

I'm feeling down (because/when/that) . . .

(e.g., "I'm feeling down because I got a bad review at my job.")

I'm gloomy . . .

I'm glum . . .

I'm unhappy . . .

I'm hurt . . .

I'm sad . . .

I'm dejected . . .

I'm depressed . . .

I'm grief-stricken . . .

I'm despondent . . .

Give Anxiety a Voice

I'm concerned (because/when/that) . . .

(e.g., "I'm concerned because I have a huge presentation to give at work.")

I'm uneasy . . .

I'm apprehensive . . .

I'm dismayed . . .

I have misgivings . . .

I'm worried . . .

I'm alarmed . . .

I'm distressed . . .

I'm afraid . . .

I'm terrified . . .

Give Guilt a Voice

I'm apologetic (because/when/that) . . .

(e.g., "I'm apologetic because I worked late again and missed dinner with my family.")

I'm contrite . . .

I'm regretful . . .

I'm remorseful . . .

I'm feeling self-reproach . . .

Give Shame a Voice

I'm abashed (because/when/that) . . .

(e.g., "I'm abashed that I ate an entire pizza by myself.")

I'm flustered . . .

I'm embarrassed . . .

I'm feeling degraded . . .

I'm mortified . . .

Give Loneliness a Voice

I'm feeling empty (because/when/that) . . .

(e.g., "I feel empty when my family doesn't visit me.")

I'm feeling alone . . .

I'm feeling isolated . . .

I'm feeling abandoned . . .

I'm feeling rejected . . .

Give Helplessness a Voice

I'm dependent (because/when/that) . . .

(e.g., "I'm dependent because I rely on my parents to pay my bills.")

I'm defenseless . . .

I'm powerless . . .

I'm weak . . .

I'm vulnerable . . .

❊ ❊ ❊

As you can see in this chapter, emotions are often the driving force behind bingeing. When you are experiencing uncomfortable feelings such as anger, sadness, anxiety, loneliness, guilt, shame, or helplessness, you may be tempted to ignore those feelings and instead focus your attention on food. Think about what types of foods you tend to binge on and what feelings you may be having in that moment. Also think about the way you talk about your body. Do you often say things like, "I feel fat" or "I ate so much my stomach hurts"? As counterintuitive as it may sound, the only way to get rid of emotions is to actually feel them. By expressing and processing what's going on inside, those feelings evaporate and you no longer feel that urge to binge.

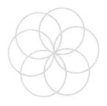

CHAPTER 3

Make Peace with Food . . . and Yourself

Imagine sitting down for a meal and eating exactly what you want, savoring each bite, and stopping when you're satisfied. Not only do you enjoy the food but you also don't have a single moment of regret afterward. That may sound impossible, but I promise you that it's not. One of the members of my online program, Kick the Diet Habit, wrote to thank me for helping her to completely transform her relationship with food. She said, "I was at a restaurant today with some friends and realized that the bread in the bread basket was nearly gone, and it never even crossed my mind to eat any. I'm seriously a free woman. I am allowing myself to eat whatever I want . . . and starting to not want or need it. I am being so kind to myself, and my confidence is through the roof. I felt so powerful. This program is working to free me!"

Another member wrote, "My life was crazy and things were out of control. I didn't have a good way to cope with problems, so I overate, and overate, and overate. I blamed myself for every bingeing episode. I knew that deeper down, I wasn't struggling with ice cream or brownies." She said that my message helped her discover the truth about not just her eating struggles but also her personal struggles. She went on to tell me, "I understand myself more than ever, and I am empowered to take control of my life, my body, and my eating."

Now it's your turn to create a peaceful and easy relationship with food. And, as you have already seen, *it's not about willpower.* You've started cracking the code to emotional eating. Now that you know what's going on inside, I'm going to teach you some new ways to respond to yourself when you're upset instead of eating. You're going to learn how to ditch your inner critic, lose the fat talk, and be a real friend to yourself.

TURN YOUR INNER CRITIC INTO A FRIEND

This is a crucial step that really helped my client Emily. When she came to see me, Emily had gained and lost twenty pounds more times than she could count. She calculated that she had gained and lost at least two hundred pounds in total since she went on her first diet at age ten. She joked that she "always found those lost pounds."

In other areas of her life, Emily was doing pretty well. She worked as a literary agent, lived in the Hollywood Hills, and had a group of really good friends. She was successful in every area except one: her weight. One day she started the session by announcing, "I'm feeling really bad about my body." A few nights earlier she had been at a party, having a great time, and suddenly she was drawn to the dessert table, which was full of cake, cookies, and brownies.

She felt like some invisible force was pulling her toward sugar. She compared it to the scene in the original *Star Wars* when the Death Star pulls in the *Millennium Falcon*. (For those of you who don't know *Star Wars*, the Death Star has this crazy gravitational force that pulls spacecraft into it, and they cannot do anything to resist.)

That's how Emily felt about brownies. The dessert table was the Death Star and she was helpless against it. She started eating brownies and then cake. She could not stop. Embarrassed, and thinking that people were watching her, she snuck a few brownies into a napkin and hid them in her pocket. She went into the bathroom to eat them in private. She stood at the bathroom sink, stuffing brownies into her mouth, crying and barely even tasting anything.

So what kind of mood do you think Emily was in, given that she was eating brownies and cake? If you're thinking that she was feeling empty and lonely, you're absolutely right.

She said, "It was horrible. Afterward I told myself, 'You're so disgusting. You have no willpower and you're completely out of control and gross.'"

I asked Emily what was going on right before she was pulled toward the dessert table. She had been having a good time until her ex-boyfriend Henry showed up with his new girlfriend, who was very thin. Emily didn't seem fazed by this.

She told me, "It's okay. What happened with Henry is ancient history. We're all good now."

Then she said, "I feel so gross and disgusting. I hate my body."

Feeling bad about her body was Emily's way of expressing and distracting from other "bad" feelings: Seeing her ex with someone new was painful, even though she tried to convince herself she was fine with the breakup. Emily felt "empty" and disconnected when it came to her relationships with guys, so filling up on desserts was a way of filling the emptiness inside.

By eating until she was stuffed and in physical pain, she converted her emotional pain to physical pain. What Emily needed was a different way to respond to herself when she was upset. She had to learn to speak differently to (and about) herself. Emily didn't realize how mean and dismissive she was to herself. I explained that thoughts lead to emotions, which in turn lead to behaviors. By speaking to herself in a harsh way, she felt bad—and then ate for comfort and distraction.

"I'm so used to doing what I do, I don't even know I'm doing it," she told me.

> "Changing the way you talk to yourself is extremely powerful."

The first step is to notice the way you talk to yourself. It's bad enough when someone else says hurtful things; it's even worse when you're saying mean things to yourself. Changing the way you talk to yourself is extremely powerful. There's a wonderful quote by body image expert Marcia Hutchinson: "If you talked to your friends the way you talk to your body, you'd have no friends left."

To break free from binge eating, be sure to talk to yourself the same way you talk to your friends. If you wouldn't say it to a friend, child, or loved one, don't say it to yourself. The next time you want to dive into a gallon of ice cream or open a giant bag of potato chips, be curious. Instead of berating yourself, ask yourself, "Why do I want to eat this? What's going on with me?" Use the Food-Mood Formula to figure out why you want to eat. Then be supportive and reassuring to yourself. If that sounds like a skill you haven't mastered, don't worry. I've developed some specific strategies to turn that inner critic into a friend.

Me, Myself, and I

Remember how Emily said to herself as she was eating brownies, "*You* are so disgusting. *You* have no willpower? *You're* completely out of control and gross?" Think about the way you talk to yourself. Maybe it's something along these lines:

- *You're not good enough.*
- *You're never going to lose weight.*
- *You're a complete failure.*

Using the pronoun "you" when you're referring to yourself means that you're using the second person. And that usually means that your inner critic is in charge of your thoughts. That critic is horrible—it makes you feel bad, and you know what? You just might be eating to escape your own mean voice. When I asked Emily to say "I am completely gross," she couldn't do it. She said it felt really harsh. And she was right.

"YOU" VERSUS "I"

Why don't you give it a try? Think of a couple of harsh phrases you say to yourself on a regular basis, or use the three examples above. Find a quiet place where you can be alone. Now, one at a time, say them out loud, first with the "you" inner critic voice, followed by the "I" voice. You can also try repeating these statements to yourself in front of a mirror. Do you find it harder when you make these statements in the first person?

Be a Friend to Yourself

Think about your very best friend in the world or someone you care about deeply. Now, imagine that person is feeling upset. Maybe she had a fight with her husband or a bad day at work. Perhaps your friend received some bad news or is exasperated with her kids. Do you say, "Oh, you're upset? Here, have some ice cream. Have some cookies. Or, eat this pizza until you feel sick." Probably not. The idea of that may seem ridiculous when it's about someone else. The best thing to say is something like, "I'm so sorry. That's really tough. How can I help?" Practice doing that for yourself. Be a friend to yourself.

First validate what you're feeling and then acknowledge it. Remind yourself that you won't always feel this way. And then ask yourself what you need to feel better. Think of the acronym VARY:

- **Validate:** *Recognize and accept what you're feeling, without judgment or apology.*
- **Acknowledge:** *Affirm the importance of what you're feeling.*
- **Reassure:** *Put yourself at ease and remind yourself that you're not always going to feel this way.*
- **Yourself:** *That's you! What do you need to feel better?*

Let's use the example of Luciana, who had to give a presentation at work. She didn't love public speaking, even to her colleagues whom she knew well. Still, she gathered her courage and gave the presentation. Everything was going well until someone on the team pointed out a mistake. Until that moment, Luciana had no idea that she'd made any errors. She was mortified by the experience. As soon as her colleague pointed out the mistake, Luciana felt her face flush red with embarrassment. She couldn't wait for the meeting to finish. As soon as it was over, she headed to the vending machine for a candy bar. She stared at the selection of candy and snacks.

At that moment the VARY acronym popped into her mind. She decided she had nothing to lose, so she gave it a try. "Of course I feel embarrassed and upset [validation]," Luciana thought. "Anyone in my position would feel this way [acknowledgment], but I'm not always going to feel this way [reassurance]. I'm certainly not the only one who's ever made a mistake, and it doesn't happen very often. I'm going to feel better tomorrow, if not sooner."

Luciana realized she already felt a little better. She thought about getting a chocolate bar but decided against it. She walked away from the vending machine without candy. The sweet response she gave to herself instead had done the trick. Like Luciana, when you honor what's going on with you and respond with kindness, it's going to feel better than calling yourself names, and you're less likely to eat for comfort.

Take Care with Your Tone

The same words can feel very different depending on what tone you use. This idea was really underscored by one of my patients, Gina, who said that she tried talking to herself and it didn't help. Gina assured me that she used all the right words but felt absolutely no different afterward. I asked her to repeat exactly what she had said, in the same way she had said it. In a flat, unemotional tone, she said, "I'm all right. This won't last. It will be okay."

Well, it was no surprise to me that Gina didn't feel better. She certainly could not expect to cheer anyone up by speaking in that way. She sounded like she was at a funeral. I suggested she inject more warmth and compassion into her voice. As an example, I repeated exactly what she had just said, only my tone was kind and reassuring. "You're all right," I said with warmth and kindness. "This won't last. It will be okay."

The same words sound completely different when you use a different tone. A soothing tone can feel like a verbal hug. When you soothe yourself with comforting words, you won't eat for comfort.

GO ON A WORD DIET

Decades ago comedian George Carlin talked about the seven words no one could say on television. He got people thinking about the way we view culture and language. Words can be extremely powerful, and they affect our experience of ourselves and the world.

I imagine that you're probably familiar with the expression "Sticks and stones may break my bones, but words can never hurt me." I completely and absolutely disagree. Broken bones can mend and be almost like new again. Words cause pain that never heals. Words weigh heavily on you. It's bad enough when someone else says hurtful things, but what about the way you talk to yourself? Here are seven words to eliminate from your vocabulary. If you want to lose weight, drop these words and see what happens.

1. Fat

"You aren't fat. You have fat. You also have fingernails. You aren't fingernails."

I don't know who originally said this, but I'd like to hug him or her. Fat talk means saying mean things about your body—or about other people's bodies. All it does is make you feel bad. Once when I was trying on some clothes in a department store, I could hear the women in the dressing room next to me talking about their bodies.

One said, "Look, I don't even have abs anymore, I have rolls. I could hide small children in my stomach rolls."

The other one retorted, "You think you're bad? I look like I *ate* a small child."

"No, you look great, but I'm a planet."

These women were talking about themselves as if they were circus freaks. Just between you and me, the more they talked, the more curious I became. I left the dressing room at the same time they were coming out of theirs. And you know what? They were two healthy, attractive, normal-looking women in their thirties. Trust me, neither one of them looked as if they were about to go into orbit.

Just a few minutes after this happened, I was waiting in line to pay for the fabulous new dress I had just tried on. A group of teenage girls behind me were trash-talking some other girl named Angelica. They were saying things like, "I don't know what that dude sees in Angelica. She's such a cow."

Another girl nodded. "Like, total whale."

Shocking, isn't it? In the space of about fifteen minutes, I heard women and girls refer to themselves or others as planets, cows, and whales. What is up with this fat talk? Fat talk makes you feel bad about yourself or others, and it reduces you (pardon the expression) to body parts. We are more than body parts. That goes for men as well as women. Keep in mind a meme I once saw on Instagram:

"If he's only interested in your legs, breasts, or thighs, send him to KFC."

Cute! When it comes to being objectified, men are not the main problem. Lots of women objectify themselves, thinking that the person in the mirror is the only one who matters. We've got to stop that. We have to start being nicer to ourselves.

You're so much more than the person in the mirror. The size of your stomach or thighs doesn't define you. What defines you is the size of your intellect, the size of your compassion, not the size of your jeans. Count the number of friends you have, not the number on the scale. Also, put a moratorium on discussing body size and shape. Stop talking about your size. Try it, just for a day. Image what you'd be thinking about or saying if you couldn't say negative things about your body. If you couldn't say anything bad about your body, what would be on your mind? Think about whether any of the following issues resonate with you right now:

- *Maybe you're having some problems at work.*
- *Maybe you're worried about your kids. Are you upset with them?*
- *Could you be mad at your husband, wife, boyfriend, or girlfriend?*
- *Are you concerned about someone in your life?*
- *Do you miss someone who's moved away or passed away?*
- *Could you be dissatisfied with some aspect of your life?*

Fat talk keeps you turning on yourself and it distracts you from some other difficult thoughts and emotions that need your attention. J. K. Rowling, the creator of the Harry Potter books, once wrote, "'Fat' is usually the first insult a girl throws at another girl when she wants to hurt her. I mean, is 'fat' really the worst thing a human being can be? Is 'fat' worse than 'vindictive', 'jealous', 'shallow', 'vain', 'boring' or 'cruel'? Not to me; but then, you might retort, what do I know about the pressure to be skinny? I'm not in the business of being judged on my looks, what with being a writer and earning my living by using my brain. . . . "

She told the story of how she went to the British Book awards, where she bumped into a woman she hadn't seen in a few years, and the woman said, "You've lost a lot of weight since the last time I saw you!" They were the first words out of her mouth.

The last time they saw each other, J. K. had just had a baby. She says, "What I felt like saying was, 'I've produced my third child and my sixth novel since I last saw you. Aren't either of those things more important, more interesting, than my size?' But no—my waist looked smaller! Forget the kid and the book: finally, something to celebrate!"

She went on to note that she has two daughters "who will have to make their way in this skinny-obsessed world," and it worried her, because she didn't want them to be "empty-headed, self-obsessed, emaciated clones." She would rather "they were independent, interesting, idealistic, kind, opinionated, original, funny —a thousand things, before 'thin.'"

As she said, quite colorfully, "I'd rather they didn't give a gust of stinking Chihuahua flatulence whether the woman standing next to them has fleshier knees than they do. Let my girls be Hermiones, rather than Pansy Parkinsons."

We tend to see the evidence we look for—in others and in ourselves. If you look for evidence that your body is gross and disgusting, you will absolutely find it. But if you look for evidence that there are parts of you that are beautiful, you will find it. Do you like your eyes, your smile, your height? Reframe the negative thought. Maybe your thighs aren't huge; maybe they're strong enough to get you where you want to go.

My friend Linda nursed her twins for more than a year, quite a feat of endurance. She was left with what she called "National Geographic boobs." Yet Linda was proud of those National Geographic boobs. Her body fed her children, and that was something she felt really good about. I love her perspective of positivity.

The way you talk about yourself—the way you talk about your body—affects the way you feel about yourself. When you are mean to yourself, you feel bad. When you feel bad, you eat for comfort.

Losing weight takes time, but you know what? You can drop the fat talk right this minute.

2. Can't

As Henry Ford famously once said, "Whether you think you can, or think you can't, you're right." The phrase "I can . . ." brings to mind possibility, things that can happen, good things, positive things. Consider these possibilities:

- *I can do this.*
- *I can be happy.*
- *I can have a good day, a good life.*
- *I can get this job.*
- *I can meet someone wonderful.*
- *I can have a good and happy life.*

That makes you feel optimistic and hopeful, and then you feel good. Put a "not" at the end of the word "can," or make it a contraction, and you have "cannot" or "can't," and that will instantly change your mood. Have you ever said anything along the lines of the following?:

- *I can't eat that.*
- *I can't lose weight.*
- *I can't stay on my eating plan.*
- *I can't take care of myself.*

If so, then you're setting yourself up to feel depressed and hopeless. Eliminate the word "can't" from your vocabulary (unless it's something like, "I can't be mean to myself because I don't deserve it.").

As a small child I loved a book titled *The Little Engine That Could*. It's about an engine that's asked to do something impossible—pull a train up a mountain. The little engine had a mantra: "I think I can." And as he slowly moved up the mountain, he said over and over, "I think I can, I think I can, I think I can . . . "

And against all odds, he does. Whatever challenges you encounter in your life, your success depends a lot on your attitude. If you tell yourself that you can do something, if you encourage yourself and believe in yourself, you're a lot more likely to reach your goal.

Remember, you've got this. You CAN do it!

3. Dumb/Stupid/Idiot

Dumb means lacking intelligence or good judgment. Stupid means lacking ordinary quickness of mind. Idiot means lacking basic ordinary reasoning. These words are often used interchangeably because they all essentially have the same meaning. As in "I can't believe I went off my diet. I'm such an idiot." Or "I feel so stupid for not knowing that my boyfriend was cheating on me." Or "I feel so dumb because my vocabulary isn't what it should be."

If a friend said, "I can't believe I ate all those cookies," what would you say to your friend? Would you say, "What's with you and the cookies, you idiot?"

Gosh, I hope not. More likely you'd say, "Hey, don't beat yourself up. Why do you think you ate those cookies? What's going on? Talk to me."

The next time you're beating yourself up over what you ate, what you weigh, your lack of exercise, or anything along those lines, ask yourself what you'd say to a friend who was telling you the same thing (assuming, of course, that you're nice to your friends). Again, if you wouldn't say it to a friend, or to a child, then don't say it to yourself.

The next time you insult your own intelligence, remember what makes you smart. Maybe you have book smarts, street smarts, or you're good at reading people. Perhaps you love to read or you can't get enough of politics. I'm sure there's something about your life that will remind you that you're not dumb or stupid or an idiot.

One day a patient said to me, "Dr. Nina, you're being too literal. When I call myself 'stupid,' I know I'm not actually stupid. It's just an expression."

Consciously knowing that you're just using an expression doesn't take away from the impact that may have on your self-esteem. Even if you know you're not stupid, another part of your mind is taking in what you're saying. If you're calling yourself names, you're bullying yourself. Being mean to yourself makes you feel bad. The next thing you know, you're eating the entire contents of your kitchen to manage that pain. On the other hand, being kind, reassuring, and supportive leads to feeling good, freeing you to make healthy, smart food choices.

4. Normal

I once saw an Instagram post depicting a girl and her mom folding laundry. The girl asks, "What is normal?"

The mother says, "It's just a setting on the dryer, honey."

According to the dictionary, normal means "conforming to a standard; usual, typical, or expected." Obviously there are some standards of behavior and ethics in our society that are expected, and typical, and behavior outside of that isn't normal. Yet many of us wonder if our thoughts, emotions, beliefs, ideas, and wishes are normal. The answer is that it's subjective and relative.

I know someone who was raised in an orthodox religious community. She began to question the Bible, something that was not acceptable in her church. In that community she was different from others and definitely not *normal*. She found a more flexible religious community in which questioning and debating the Bible was encouraged. That religious community fit her like a glove. Her intellectual curiosity, the very thing that was devalued in the previous community, was now considered an asset. If you feel like a square peg trying to fit into a round hole, there's nothing wrong with you. The problem is that you're trying to make something fit when it doesn't. Instead, find a "square hole."

Most of us are familiar with Hans Christian Andersen's tale of the ugly duckling. A mother duck hatches a bunch of eggs, but the last one, the biggest, is slow to hatch and he is large and ugly, not at all like the other ducklings. His duckling brothers and sisters mock him. They wish the farmhouse cat would get him. His mother wishes he'd never been born. Finally the duckling runs away. During the harsh, cold, and lonely winter that follows, he encounters all kinds of dangers.

One day, when he cannot bear another day of misery, he comes across a flock of swans. He imagines that being killed by swans is preferable to the horrors he has survived. Bending his head to the water, he waits for the swans to finish him off. When he glimpses his reflection, he is astonished. He is no longer an ugly duckling. He has become what he actually has been all along: a graceful and beautiful swan. The other swans accept him and welcome him into their fold.

That story has held different meanings for me at various phases of my life. When I was a child who didn't fit in with the rest of my family, it gave me hope that one day I could find another family where I fit in. When I was a teenager, it gave me hope that I would grow out of my gawky, awkward, ugly phase and someday be beautiful, someday fit in. Later it served as an allegory about inner strength, survival, and tenacity. It's also a reminder that what is considered normal is highly subjective. What's normal for some people isn't for others. Ultimately this story is about appreciating who you are and trusting that with the right community of friends and loved ones, you will flourish. Try not to get so caught up in words like *normal* that if you don't feel you fit in with society's standards, you turn to bingeing to comfort yourself.

5. Ridiculous

According to the dictionary, the word "ridiculous" means "deserving or inviting derision or mockery; absurd." This definition is problematic because the notion of what is ridiculous can be subjective. It's definitely ridiculous to ask a homeless person for some money because that makes no sense. It's also ridiculous to think that pigs might sprout wings because that's not going to happen.

Yet that's not how the word is usually used. One of my patients told her father that she disliked a movie that he liked, and he told her, "Don't be ridiculous. That was a terrific film." Since he'd really enjoyed the movie, he couldn't tolerate the idea that his daughter had her own mind and that she held separate opinions. He couldn't stand that she was her own person and not an extension of him, so he labeled her ridiculous whenever they disagreed. Expressing what you think or feel, or what you want or need, is never ridiculous.

Unfortunately, when we are made to feel ridiculous by other people, it can cause us to bury our emotions. And how do we do that? By bingeing on food to avoid feeling our emotions.

6. Should

How often do you find yourself using the word "should"—especially when it comes to food or your eating habits? I bet if you counted how many times you thought or said this word with regard to yourself, you'd be surprised. Maybe you often find yourself thinking one of the following thoughts:

- *I should not do that.*
- *I should not have eaten that.*
- *I shouldn't eat that.*
- *I shouldn't want that.*
- *I should be better at this.*
- *I should get a better job.*
- *I should have a boyfriend/girlfriend.*

As a professor of mine used to say, "Don't should on yourself!" The word "should" causes us to direct anxiety, sadness, anger, and distress toward ourselves. Those feelings may be so powerful that we use food to cope. Instead, be interested in your thoughts/ emotions rather than judgmental. Instead of "should-ing" on yourself, be curious. The more you ask questions, the more likely you are to find answers.

7. But

"But" is another word that can feel disempowering. Think about the following statements:

- *"I got that promotion, **but** that was just because I worked really hard. If I were really smart, I wouldn't have had to work so hard."*
- *"I feel good today. **But** that could change tomorrow."*
- *"I did my best time in that half marathon. **But** other people are still faster than I am."*

What do you notice about the impact of the word "but" in those sentences? In each case, it totally negates anything positive. When you eliminate this word from your vocabulary, you're left with: "I got a promotion. I feel good today. I did my best time in that half marathon."

That feels a lot better. No buts about it.

As you can see, the way you talk to yourself has a profound effect on your well-being, which is why I suggest you eliminate these seven words. When you feel good, wondering what you're going to eat will be more about fueling your body and enjoying your meals, instead of entering a battlefield of guilt and self-recrimination every time you eat. Take off the weight of the word, starting now!

CLEAN UP YOUR VOCABULARY

Look back at the seven words in this section. How often do you use them? Do you find yourself using certain words more than others? Keep track for a day or two. Most of us have our phones with us all the time, so make a quick note whenever you notice yourself using any of these words. Once you become more aware of it, it will be easier to break the habit.

DECLARE A TRUCE WITH NUMBERS

"I hate shopping for jeans." That's the beginning of a Special K commercial in which several women are talking about how painful, depressing, and heartbreaking it is to shop for jeans. They go shopping and discover a store where the jeans have no sizes. They find the jeans that fit by using a measuring tape that has no numbers. Instead the measurements are: charismatic, radiant, fabulous, stunning, confident, strong, and awesome.

That's a measuring tape we all need!

If you're relying on numbers to define you—the size of your body, the size of your jeans, the number on the scale—then you're limiting your total sense of self to your physical self and ignoring everything else that's important. What about your emotional, intellectual, relational self? What about your values?

Do you know anyone who's really terrific? I'm guessing that you do. Take a moment and consider what makes that person so cool and amazing. Is it the size of her jeans? The gap between her thighs? Her weight?

No, of course not! What makes a person awesome is integrity, intelligence, kindness, warmth, and spirit, to name just a few qualities. You can't weigh awesome because it's a "way" of being, not a number.

I once asked thousands of my Facebook followers to name the most awesome person they knew, and I received a range of answers. Some said their mom or dad was the most awesome person they knew, and described them as "always there for others" or said they "put their family first" or that they "know how to cheer people up and never judge."

Others said their brothers and sisters were awesome because of their confidence, optimism, positivity, and the fact that they were good role models. They could count on their siblings to be there no matter what, unconditionally.

A lot of people thought their friends were the most awesome people they knew. They described their friends as understanding, accepting, fun-loving, intelligent, open-minded, happy, positive, friendly, and available. They also used words such as loyal, responsible, creative, strong, generous, and loving. Others mentioned their therapists and their bosses, and they talked about qualities such as persistence, tenacity, fearlessness, speaking up, and doing the right thing.

No one said, "My friend Blah-Blah-Blah is awesome because she has no cellulite." Or "My friend So-and-So has six-pack abs."

You probably wouldn't like your friends better if they lost weight. You wouldn't say, "If only my best friend would drop a few pounds. She'd be so much nicer." The very thought is absurd. You like your friends because they're good listeners, they make you laugh, they're there for you, you have fun together, and you have a lot in common. It's time to appreciate yourself the way you appreciate other people in your life. If those measures aren't even a blip on the radar of your self-esteem, it's time to find a new definition of self-worth.

Think about this: Are you there for others? Are you accepting and nonjudgmental? Are you understanding, fun-loving, intelligent, open-minded, happy, positive, friendly, and available? Loyal, responsible, creative, strong, generous, or loving? Persistent, tenacious? Do you always try to do the right thing?

"No matter how much weight you're trying to lose, I want you to feel good about yourself during the process."

If any of those qualities describe you, then guess what? You're awesome. No matter how much weight you're trying to lose, I want you to feel good about yourself during the process. Don't make your self-worth contingent on some magical number on the scale. You can feel good about yourself even when you want to lose weight—even while you're losing weight.

WHAT MAKES YOU AWESOME?

Take a few moments to write down five positive characteristics/qualities about yourself that have nothing to do with your weight. A bonus challenge is to ask your loved ones what they consider your best qualities. This can be a vulnerable exercise but ultimately very rewarding.

BABY YOURSELF

Heather was a new mom, and she was always trying to figure out what her baby was feeling. Whenever the baby cried, Heather tried to discover what was wrong. She wondered if the baby was tired. Or possibly hungry. Did she need a diaper change? Was she crying because she wanted to be held? In contrast to Heather, who tried to uncover exactly why her baby was crying, some mothers respond to every cry with food. The baby may be tired, hungry, wet, or just cranky, but the response is the same: The baby gets a bottle or a breast. This may not seem like a big deal, but it's actually the starting point of emotional eating.

Imagine this experience from a baby's perspective: You're sleepy and need to nap, so you cry. Mom comes over right away, but instead of soothing you and helping you nap, she provides a bottle. When this happens over and over, you learn that your need for rest will be resolved with food. You may even start to confuse the need for rest with hunger. If this happens repeatedly, you may even feel hungry when you're actually tired. As I watched Heather respond to her daughter, I reflected on how nice it would be if more people babied themselves. If you struggle with food, you may be hostile to your basic needs, whether for food, sleep, love, connection, or comfort.

By learning strategies to "baby" yourself, recognizing and validating your needs instead of condemning them, you feel better. When you feel good, you won't turn to food as a way of symbolically meeting your needs. Below are some steps you can take to do exactly that.

Step 1: Get Comfortable with Your Needs and Wants

Aesop was a slave in ancient Greece whose stories have a lot of significance in our modern age. One of Aesop's fables involves a fox who is trotting along the road, going wherever foxes go, when he suddenly stumbles across a grapevine. Bunches of plump grapes hang tantalizingly out of reach. The fox does everything in his power to reach those grapes, but it's useless. After jumping, climbing, and leaping, it's all too clear to the fox that there is no way of reaching those grapes.

"They are probably sour, anyway," the fox sniffs, trotting away.

This illustrates the way we sometimes deal with disappointment when our needs aren't met. When our needs aren't met, or aren't adequately met, we may shrug and say that the thing we needed was no good. There is a difference between "having needs" and "being needy." If you're human, then, like it or not, you have needs. All of us have basic needs for food, water, and shelter, and we have other needs: for love, affection, connection, attention, and a sense of meaningfulness in our lives. We need emotional support from others because we are social, and we need to both give and receive caring, understanding, companionship, and all kinds of other types of help. But sometimes we have trouble accepting that we need help, as illustrated in the example below.

John came back from Home Depot with a truck loaded with supplies. He and his wife had just bought their first house, and they were doing a lot of home improvement projects. John started lugging heavy bags of supplies and big cans of paint toward the house. His wife immediately offered to help.

John didn't say, "Thanks, honey. Can you take this bag?"

Instead John snapped, "I've got this."

His wife tried again, saying, "C'mon, let me help," and again he refused.

In fact, he raised his voice a bit. "I told you, I can do it myself!"

When John was a child and needed help with his homework, his mother always told him to ask his father. And his father thought John should learn to figure it out for himself. When John had issues at school with bullies or problems with friends, or even when he needed help making toy models (he made Star Trek models) his father told him, "You can handle this yourself."

In response to all John's needs for help, guidance, and reassurance, his parents advised him to be self-sufficient. He took this to mean that his needs were too much for his parents and began equating "having needs" with "being needy." He couldn't let anyone help him—not even his wife—because that would make him feel needy and weak.

After he put away the supplies from Home Depot, John went into the pantry and tore open a box of Oreo cookies. He crammed cookies into his mouth. Later he apologized to his wife for snapping at her. He was upset at himself for doing that. And he was mad at himself for scarfing down Oreos. All that self-recrimination distracted from his inner conflict about needing help.

John realized he could have used some help. The bags were heavy. Rationally he knew there was no shame in getting help, and he felt foolish for reacting so strongly. Another side of John, the part that identified with his father, felt weak for wanting or needing any kind of help—especially from his wife. He could hear his father's voice in his head: *What kind of a man are you, needing help from your wife?* His childhood had conditioned him to prize independence and view help as weakness. His solution was cookies, which distanced him from the humiliation of needing something from another person, a situation he had constantly experienced with his dad. In this way John replaced the shame of having needs with the shame of eating cookies.

Many people think they're "needy" when they actually have natural, normal human needs. They struggle with wanting more from other people, fearing that they will be "too much" or that others will reject them if they express themselves in an authentic manner.

If you cannot trust that others will be there for you, then it might feel too risky to be hungry for love and intimacy, to need attention and connection. If those needs aren't met, or aren't met consistently, or if you're shamed for expressing needs, it's humiliating. That's when "having needs" feels like you're "being needy."

There are three ways to respond to your needs:

1) Acknowledge them.

2) Meet them.

3) Come to terms with unmet needs.

Consider the example of Carolyn, who returned from a mountain-biking trip with her boyfriend. She opened the hatch of her SUV, and as she struggled to lift out the heavy bike, her boyfriend hurried toward her, offering to help.

Carolyn declined. "I can do it myself," she said.

She managed the burden of the heavy bike, rejecting all her boyfriend's attempts to assist. With great difficulty she struggled to get the bike out of the vehicle and wheeled it into the garage, leaving her boyfriend bewildered and upset.

Carolyn winced at the memory. "I couldn't let him help me. I can't let anyone help me do something that I can do myself."

She didn't know why she'd had such a strong reaction. She just couldn't stand letting anyone do something for her if she could do it herself. She described the feeling as that sensation you get when you hold opposing magnets together.

"What's wrong with letting someone help you?" I asked.

She recoiled, looking stricken. "I can't. That would make me weak."

Carolyn had a difficult time recognizing that her wish for help was absolutely normal. People who are conflicted about their needs often feel weak for having them. They feel selfish whenever they try to meet their needs. No one had ever shamed Carolyn for having needs, but she remembered how her uncle responded when her brother needed something. Her uncle called her brother horrible names: Sissy boy. Girl. Baby. Carolyn had made it a point not to do anything that would make her uncle talk to her that way.

Leadership coach Marcia Reynolds suggests looking at needs from a new angle. As she said in a 2015 *Psychology Today* article, "My need for attention helps me to succeed as a writer, teacher and public speaker. My need for recognition drives my desire to do good work. My need for control helps me take charge of projects and run a successful business."

Once you identify what your needs actually are, it's time to take care of yourself and meet those needs. If you're lonely, spend time with friends. If you need a hug, get one—or give one. If you're angry, talk to someone about it, or take a kickboxing class to relieve the physical intensity of anger. If you're sad, allow yourself to cry.

Perhaps you're heard the expression "What you resist will persist." If you don't deal with the fact of not getting what you needed earlier in your life, you're likely to unconsciously repeat old patterns in an attempt to get those needs from the past met in the present. Or you may shift your need from something to do with people onto food. We'll be exploring this in more detail later on in the book.

IDENTIFY YOUR NEEDS AND WANTS

Make a list of your top three needs. Now make a list of your top three wants. How are you meeting those needs and wants? What can you do to ensure you don't ignore them? Are there ways that you can better express them or get closer to obtaining them?

Step 2: Develop an Appetite for Life

One of the most poignant moments in the classic novel and movie *Oliver Twist* occurs when little Oliver bravely steps up to the overseer to ask for more gruel. Oliver is nine years old and has already suffered a lot. After his mother dies in the street, he's consigned to a workhouse, where he and the other boys are starved.

"Please, sir, I want some more."

The overseer, a heavy man who knows nothing of starvation, starts beating poor Oliver with a ladle. For Oliver, asking for more food was seen as tantamount to a crime. And, for many of us, wanting more out of life is seen as greedy or unbecoming. Societal messages caution that we should be grateful for what we have. Wanting more out of life becomes a minefield of danger.

Yet wanting more is human. Zulaikha recalled spending childhood afternoons at her grandparents' house while her parents were at work. Her grandparents were immigrants who had fled war to come to the United States. They worked hard, saved every penny, and made a big deal out of being self-reliant.

When Zulaikha wanted a new toy or a new doll, they asked if it was something she *wanted* or *needed*. The message was that needing something for survival was acceptable. Simply wanting something, coveting a toy or wishing for a day at the amusement park, was frowned upon. Zulaikha felt ashamed and greedy for wanting the same things that her American classmates took for granted. At the same time that she received the message not to want frivolous things, she was invited to eat as much as she wanted. Her parents and grandparents heaped piles of food on her plate, urging her to have more. "Eat, eat, you're a growing girl."

Food was the one thing she could say she wanted more of, so Zulaikha ate more and more and more. This was the only reliable outlet where she could allow her wishes to surface, and they were all displaced onto food. Accept that you may have "wants" in life and that you don't need to repress them with food. Go ahead—have an appetite for life.

FILLING THE EMPTY SPACE

When we feel deprived, food isn't the only way that we unconsciously enact our need for more. You've probably heard the term "retail therapy." People often shop when they're stressed or upset or sad (that's the retail part) because it makes them feel better (that's the therapy part). It's the same with food—lots of people eat for comfort or distractions. If you overspend as well as overeat, there may well be a connection between how you spend money and what's going on with food. And just as bingeing can make you feel guilty and ashamed afterward, ultimately making you feel worse, so too can overspending. How often have you returned home from a shopping spree only to regret your purchases or feel some level of guilt for spending money?

Think about the experience of zoning out, being in a different state of mind by "spacing out" or "going blank." People describe both food binges and shopping sprees in exactly the same way. There is no question that both overeating and overspending are ways of managing uncomfortable or intolerable moods. But let's go a bit deeper. Those behaviors also help you:

1) Manage emptiness and loneliness

2) Express conflicts over abundance

3) Take you away from yourself

Often you get so good at using these coping mechanisms that you don't even know what's really going on inside. One way to figure it out is to examine what you're buying. Much like the Food-Mood Formula, which correlates certain foods with certain emotions, wishes, and conflicts, taking a look at what you purchase can open a window to what's hidden. When you see more clearly, you can take action to change.

WHAT EMOTIONS ARE YOU SUPPRESSING WITH RETAIL THERAPY?

Think back to the last time you went on a shopping binge. What did you purchase? How did it make you feel? Perhaps you bought objects that take up space in your home or you filled your closet with new styles, almost as though you were trying on a new personality. When you get to the bottom of why you're buying certain items, you will stop stuffing down your emotions with retail therapy.

What Is the Empty Space?

If you buy a lot of the same thing, maybe even think of yourself as a collector, it's possible that you're symbolically filling a void. Objects take up space in our homes just as food takes up space in our stomachs.

I treated Linda for more than a year before I discovered that she had an issue with overspending as well as overeating. She just happened to mention that the day before, she had stopped herself from shopping with the same willpower she usually reserved for dieting. Linda told me she had a weakness for bedsheets.

She said, "I have no room in my house for more sheets, but I saw such a pretty set of sheets on sale and I couldn't help myself. I have a thing about sheets."

I knew that Linda lived alone in a large home that once belonged to her parents. "What do you mean, no room for sheets?"

As it turned out, Linda had more than 150 sets of sheets, which took up a lot of space. When we explored her "thing" about sheets, she said she liked new sheets because they were nice and fresh, and that was all there was to it. When we explored this further, she remembered staying at her friend's house overnight when she was a kid. During those sleepovers there was always a fresh, clean, pretty sheet on the bed. The friend's parents were loving and affectionate. Linda's parents both drank themselves into a stupor on a regular basis. They often got into physical fights, screaming and throwing things at each other. For Linda, the sheets came to represent the kind of life she wanted, the kind of relationship she craved. She couldn't have the happy family, but she could have the sheets, and the sense of happiness was always one sheet away.

I said, "Linda, it seems to me that buying all these sheets is your way of trying to connect to a sense of having a loving family."

She said, "No sheet."

Linda had a sense of humor and a fast wit. We both laughed at her joke but recognized the painful underpinnings of what Linda called her "sheet addiction." Once she identified why she felt so compelled to buy new sheets, she was able to express what she was truly hungry for and got in touch with the emptiness that no amount of sheets or food could ever fill. She had to mourn the family she had, and to process the loss of never having the kind of loving family she craved. Only then did she stop buying sheets and bingeing. She realized that she was feeling what poet Edna St. Vincent Millay called "the presence of an absence." Linda had been trying to fill the absence by stuffing her house with sheets and filling her body with food.

Is Life a Struggle?

Some people spend money on all kinds of things, finding themselves without enough funds and mounting credit card debt, barely scraping by until the next paycheck, and often on the financial edge. Some believe that it's noble to suffer, so having too much registers as wrong or greedy. For others, remaining financially dependent on family members gives them a sense of being taken care of, as if there is a financial umbilical cord that keeps them connected to other people and makes them feel loved.

Just as food sometimes represents love, so does money.

Patrice was overeducated and overqualified for her job at Trader Joe's. She had a master's degree but was barely making more than minimum wage. Underpaid and undervalued, she was constantly looking for a better job. She figured once she got that job, she'd stop living paycheck to paycheck and wouldn't have to depend on her parents for extra money.

Patrice eventually did find a better job. What do you think happened next? In a perfect world, she opened a savings account, contributed to a 401K, and breathed a sigh of relief at finding herself in a financially comfortable position. Instead Patrice bought expensive clothes, expensive groceries, and a more expensive car. She continued to live paycheck to paycheck, and her parents continued helping her make ends meet. Patrice felt guilty for getting herself into a financial mess and ate ice cream to soothe herself. It was hard for her to get in touch with her hurt and resentful feelings toward her parents for being so emotionally withholding. She denied that anger but got mad at herself for gaining weight and staying poor, instead of expressing her true feelings.

Patrice came to realize that she stayed dependent on her parents because their money was a form of love. They couldn't provide anything that resembled emotional support, but they could freely give financial support. If she didn't need their monetary help, she feared on some level she'd lose their love.

For Patrice, expressing her feelings didn't mean actually telling her parents she was upset. That wouldn't have gone well since they were incapable of hearing her. Expressing anger meant first admitting to herself that she was angry, resentful, and sad. Patrice processed her feelings and started healing. She met with a financial adviser and created a budget. In time it became easier for her to regulate both money and food, and as her bank account grew, her weight dropped.

Dressed to Impress

Do you buy a lot of clothes, shoes, or cosmetics? If so, maybe you're trying to create a different persona. Maybe clothes and appearance-related items make you feel like the person you want to be because who you are doesn't seem good enough. That's what was going on with Ariana, who admitted that she had a different wardrobe for all her different lives. She bought work clothes, weekend clothes, clothes she wore when she hung out with her artsy band friends, and clothes she wore around her family.

Ariana's clothing functioned like a costume, making her a chameleon in different situations. She didn't think that she was good enough just as herself. When she wasn't shopping for clothes, she was bingeing on food. Ariana shopped and ate to distract herself from uncomfortable thoughts and feelings. When she learned to slow down, to respond to herself in a new way—truly believing she was good enough no matter whom she was around—she was able to stop using both food and shopping as a distraction.

If you're empty and lonely, no amount of things or food will fill that void. If you're struggling with conflicts about independence or abundance, shopping and eating only provide a temporary distraction. If you don't feel comfortable with yourself, clothes, makeup, and hair products won't make you feel better about yourself—and food won't make you feel better, either.

To liberate yourself from dieting, remember the real battleground isn't eating or shopping—it's your relationship with yourself. When you fight through and resolve those conflicts, they disappear for good and so do your bingeing habits.

❋ ❋ ❋

Once you make peace with your inner critic—and the scale—you will make peace with food. Remember, words are extremely powerful, so be careful how you talk to yourself. Speak to yourself the way you would comfort a dear friend. Instead of a food diet, go on a word diet and eliminate the words fat, can't, dumb/stupid/idiot, normal, ridiculous, should, and but from your vocabulary (at least with regard to yourself!). You are so much more than a number on the scale, so when you find yourself struggling, remember that list you made earlier of all the amazing qualities that make you who you are. Learn to respond to your wants and needs instead of trying to fill an empty space with food or material items. As Dr. Seuss said, "Today you are you, that is truer than true. There is no one alive who is youer than you." Never forget that you are good enough just as you are.

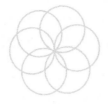

CHAPTER 4

Free Yourself from the Past—and Transform Your Present

Our past can actually have a powerful influence on our present feelings and food habits. For many of us, our first experience of love and comfort was being fed in one of our parent's arms. The desire to reconnect to this time of love and safety can make us turn to food during difficult times. The truth is that people disappoint us, hurt us, leave us, or make us angry. But unlike people, food is reliable. It can be easy to fall into a routine of soothing ourselves with food when what we really need is comfort, love, and support from another person. Often an experience in our past leads us to feel "not good enough." Unfortunately, those feelings of inadequacy can lead us to try to fill that emptiness with food.

If you were given food to help quell your feelings when you were young, you likely carried this pattern into adulthood. If you had an angry or dismissive parent, you may have learned to repress uncomfortable feelings with food. Childhood experiences affect how you relate to yourself and the world, so if your parent had a negative response to your feelings, it may have taught you to dismiss your emotions and instead eat for comfort. In this chapter we'll explore the ways in which these past experiences can manifest as food issues in adulthood, as well as how relationships from your past can often repeat in the present with authority figures such as bosses representing parents. This is not about blaming your parents—it's about explaining where these past beliefs stemmed from so that you can understand how they have affected you, release them, and move on. We'll also examine your attachment style—anxious-preoccupied, dismissive-avoidant, fearful-avoidant, or secure—as this can help illuminate your relationship with food as well.

I will help you determine if you are replacing the "food of love" with a "love of food" because you feel vulnerable and do not trust relationships. What exactly is your relationship with food? Do you love it, do you have a love-hate relationship with it, or do you hate/fear it? Your food issues can be a reflection of your deeper feelings about your intimate relationships, but you can learn how to fill yourself with meaningful connections with other people instead of filling up on food.

Finally, we'll take a look at the difference between being selfish and being selfless and you'll learn a third option: self-care. When you learn to balance your own needs, set limits, and stop people-pleasing, you will no longer need to eat as a distraction from anxiety or guilt.

WHY FOOD?

Take a moment to consider the last time you ate something to feel better. Maybe it was cookies or ice cream or a big plate of pasta. Think about whether you were physically hungry or if something else was going on. Perhaps you had a deeper hunger for something emotionally fulfilling.

Your relationship with food can be an expression of what is missing in your life. If you don't have enough of what you need, food symbolically fills the emptiness inside and provides comfort, but it's an illusory and temporary fix. Many expressions utilize food metaphors to describe a feeling of yearning: *hungry for love*, *starving for attention*, and *an appetite for life*. If there's something missing from your life, that may have to do with your relationships.

This was the case with Bettina, who was a dieting veteran by the time she was in middle school. Her pediatrician placed her on an eight-hundred-calorie-a-day weight-loss plan, and she had been dieting ever since. Each lost pound was a cause for celebration. Every time she lost weight, Bettina promised herself that she would never regain the weight, only to feel hopeless when those pounds inevitably returned. Not only did Bettina hope to lose weight once and for all, but she also wanted to get past what she called her "crazy obsession" with food. Her mind was constantly preoccupied with thoughts of food, and she had cravings that were so intense that she often felt overwhelmed.

"Why is food my thing?" lamented Bettina. "If I used crack or meth to numb myself, at least I'd be skinny."

Sadly, she was not kidding.

So why food? Many of us turn to food when we are upset, lonely, or bored because our first experience of love, safety, and bonding is connected to being fed in infancy. When you see a parent feeding a baby, you see love flowing between them. For a baby or a young child, being held in a mother's or father's arms, feeling loved and safe, is bound up with the experience of feeding. Food is experienced as love. We learn to associate food with a blissful connection to another person.

The experience of being fed becomes an experience of being loved. That's why—and this may sound a little strange at first— deep in our psyches, food actually represents people. We don't consciously think of it that way, but consider how we use the same words for both food and love. We describe relationships as *fulfilling* or *satisfying*. We talk about being *hungry for love* or say someone is *starving for attention*. Thought of in this manner, turning to food can be understood as a way of unconsciously rediscovering the experience of love and the peaceful, blissful serenity and connection of an earlier time in our lives, when safety, love, and satisfaction were bound up in feeding. When we turn to food to feel better, it's an attempt to provide an experience of soothing, comforting, or relaxing.

If you're lonely, you may not be able to find anyone to talk to you or hold you. Even if someone is there with you, that person might not respond the way you want—or may not satisfy your need for connection. People might not love you back; they might disappoint you, cheat on you, or just not be there for you.

The bottom line? People can be unpredictable, unavailable, or unreliable. Unlike people, food is always there when you need it.

Unlike people, food is always the same. Ice cream always tastes the same. Chips are chips. Cake is cake. You get the idea. Unlike people, food is predictable, available, and reliable.

WHEN DID YOU STOP FEELING "GOOD ENOUGH?"

Maybe, consciously or unconsciously, you believe something along these lines: "People can't be trusted to meet my needs consistently, so I'll have food instead. Food is always available, always consistent, and it fills up my internal emptiness." When you have satisfying and fulfilling connections, you don't need food as a substitute for people. Of course, that is much easier said than done. Just ask Zoe, who wanted to join my weekly eating disorder support group. Something always came up and she never actually made it to the group. Zoe finally confessed that she was afraid she would be, in her words, "the fattest one in the room."

This fear also affected her personal life. She wouldn't meet friends in restaurants because she was afraid she'd be the fattest one there. She didn't want to go to the gym for the same reason. She lamented her lack of willpower, and she thought her body was disgusting and gross. She was so concerned that she'd be the biggest one in the room that she stayed home. And when Zoe was home, she ate. Whether or not Zoe would have in fact been the biggest person in the room was irrelevant. Lots of people feel that way, whether they weigh 400 pounds or 140 pounds.

I asked Zoe what would happen if she actually were the biggest person in the room, whether it was my support group, the gym, the office, a restaurant, a party, or anywhere else. What then? What did she imagine people were thinking about her?

She said, "They'd think I have no willpower. They'd think I'm disgusting and gross. They wouldn't want to have anything to do with me."

Notice how that was almost word for word how Zoe described herself. She assumed people were thinking the very same harsh thoughts that she did. Without even realizing it she was projecting her own thoughts onto others, then directing those mean thoughts back at herself.

Most of us aren't psychic. We don't actually know what's going on in the minds of others. But if you imagine that people are thinking the most awful, critical, and judgmental thoughts, think about the way you relate to yourself. Consider whether the thoughts you imagine other people have about you are the same thoughts you have about yourself. Zoe realized she was afraid of something else: If she were the biggest one in the room, she thought the other group members would think they were better than she was, and she didn't want to feel inferior to them.

This fear went all the way back to Zoe's childhood, when she and her siblings were always trying to outdo the other. They competed for who got the best grades, who could eat ice cream the slowest, who could stay up the latest, and more. Not only did Zoe think the group would judge her weight, but she also imagined they would relate to her as her siblings had in the past. She didn't want to experience that kind of rivalry.

Zoe needed to develop an invisible mental shield, kind of like a *Star Wars* deflector shield. We created what we called "emotional Teflon" by considering alternative scenarios to the one Zoe had in her head. Zoe visualized the group welcoming her, relating to her, and making her feel understood. She imagined people at the gym looking at her and thinking, "Good for her, getting healthy."

I have a friend from Texas who likes to say, "Go big or go home." When you're visualizing something new and pleasant, that's the time to go big, to be an emotional heavyweight, to be a person with the biggest self-confidence and the largest sense of self. Consider what aspects of yourself—physical, intellectual, mental, emotional—you feel good about, right now, at this weight, at this stage of your life. Remember that the number on the bathroom scale doesn't define you. That scale measures only your weight, not your value as a person. Keep in mind that the size of your kindness, generosity, intelligence, and compassion is a far better measure of yourself. If other people don't see past the number on the scale, then you've got their number, so to speak. And guess what? You can delete it. When you feel good about yourself, you're far less likely to turn to food for comfort or distraction—because you don't need distraction from happiness and self-acceptance.

DO YOU FEEL "GOOD ENOUGH?"

Challenge the idea that you're not good enough as you are. Ask yourself where that idea came from in the first place. Recall a time when you didn't worry about your weight and you felt carefree and happy. Think about what has changed since that time.

COOKIES DON'T CHANGE FEELINGS

A few years ago I was at a park, watching my daughter play with her friends on the jungle gym. A few feet away from me, two toddlers—a boy and a girl—were sitting in the sand together, digging with sand toys and sifting sand, and they were completely engrossed in this activity. Suddenly the little guy climbed to his feet, clutching the shovel. He tottered on unsteady legs for a few moments, then he scampered off across the playground. The girl looked after him in confusion and burst into tears.

Her mother came running up, looking anxious. "Don't cry," she pleaded. "Don't cry. It's okay."

The girl was sobbing. After all, the little dude just took off and left her without warning (I'm sure many of us can relate to that experience of being dumped without warning), and, to make matters worse, he still had her shovel. Her tears were a natural response to hurt feelings.

Her mother urged, "Stop crying. It's okay."

Mom opened the diaper bag and started digging around inside, growing more visibly anxious as her daughter sobbed. "Shhhhhh, don't cry," she pleaded.

The girl wailed, inconsolable.

Mom pulled a box of animal crackers from the diaper bag. "Here," she said, shoving a cookie into the girl's hand. "Have a cookie."

Yikes. I really, really, really wanted to say something to that mother like, "Don't do that! Stop teaching your kid to be scared of her feelings and to use cookies for comfort." I held my tongue, but it wasn't easy. What did that toddler learn in the moment? That her feelings can make other people anxious. That she should not cry or get upset. But if she absolutely can't stop herself from crying, a cookie will help.

Afterward it occurred to me that the exchange between this mom and her daughter also mimics the internal dialogue that many people have when they get upset. It's very likely that little girl will grow up to be a woman who reaches for cookies when she feels anxious. Her experiences as a toddler will continue to be enacted through her life. She won't know why she turns to food as an adult. She won't realize that she was taught to do so and never learned any other way of coping.

> "As counterintuitive as it may seem, the only way to get rid of feelings is to actually experience and feel them."

Here's the thing: Cookies do not actually take away feelings. You can't stuff feelings down; you can't starve them away, purge them, drink them away, gamble them away, work them away, let them go, or use positive thinking to get rid of them. As you know from the previous section of this book, there's only one way to get rid of feelings. As counterintuitive as it may seem, the only way to get rid of feelings is to actually experience and feel them.

If the mother had said, "Sweetie, I know it hurts. It's painful when people leave you and take your things and you don't know why they do it," then the girl would have had a good cry and felt better.

That's how you get rid of feelings for good.

Other parents might have responded differently to the same situation. A **dismissive parent** might not even have noticed the girl was crying or may have glanced over and said, "You're okay. It's not the end of the world." In that situation the child would learn that her feelings were of no interest to others. She would be more likely to grow up and dismiss her experience, admonishing herself that it "isn't a big deal" and telling herself to get over it.

Let's imagine you go to the park and you see a little boy fall off the monkey bars. He hurts his elbow, which is skinned and raw. He runs up to his father, showing him the injury. "Dad, my elbow. It hurts so much."

Dad looks over, squints at the injury. "What are you talking about? That's barely a scratch."

Tears are running down the boy's face. "It hurts. Look, it's bleeding."

Dad says, "Don't be ridiculous—you're fine. Stop whining."

Maybe he even says, "Don't be such a baby. It's just a little scratch."

Harsh, huh? This is an example of overt dismissiveness. Or, if the first kind is pretty dismissive, I guess this is ugly dismissiveness.

In this case that boy learns that expressing pain bothers other people and that others might react to him in a scornful way. He learns that other people have no tolerance for what he's feeling— because if his dad doesn't care, why should anyone else? Whether the dismissiveness is overt or covert, it conveys the same message, which is that you don't know your own feelings and you shouldn't feel them.

An **angry parent** might snap, "Stop crying, already!" or "I'll give you something to cry about!" An angry response teaches children that their feelings upset others, and the best way to avoid anger is to keep feelings to themselves.

A **supportive parent** would say, "Of course you're upset. It's okay to cry it out. Your feelings are hurt." This last response is the ideal way to respond to children, and it's the best way to respond to ourselves when we are upset.

Think about how your own parents responded to your feelings when you were a child. Can you remember any particular scenarios when they may have been dismissive or angry? How did that make you feel? Were you ever given food as a way to silence those feelings? Think about how this may or may not continue to affect you in the present day and learn how to be a supportive parent to yourself when you need it.

DISMISSING EMOTIONAL PAIN

The key to changing your relationship with food is to change your relationship with your feelings. When you can be supportive of yourself, instead of responding with anxiety, dismissal, or anger, you will be less likely to turn to food.

When you're upset, do you tell yourself one of the following things?

- *Don't worry, it could be a lot worse.*
- *You have a lot to be grateful for.*
- *Look on the bright side. This isn't so bad.*

That may not seem dismissive, but it is. Although it appears to be nice and reassuring, it's just a sweet way of discounting what's bothering you. To stop overeating you have to deal with what you feel.

This is harder than it sounds. Despite everything I know about responding to feelings, I don't always get it right. I remember a time when I picked up my youngest daughter from school and saw her running around with her friends, laughing, playing, and having fun. Suddenly my daughter fell and scraped her knee on the gravel. She got up, clutching her knee, which was bleeding.

She ran up to me, crying, "Look what happened! It's bleeding. It hurts."

I looked at her knee and saw it was raw and scraped but not bleeding too badly. And then I made my first mistake. I said, "Oh, that's not so bad."

She started crying harder, tears streaming down her face. "It hurts, mama. It *hurts*."

That's when I made my second mistake. I repeated, "It's not that bad. And look, you only skinned *one* knee. Just think how much it would hurt if you skinned both of them."

My daughter kept crying. I kept saying the wrong things, telling her, "Let's get a Band-Aid on that. You're fine, it's okay."

My daughter wailed, "But it HURTS."

And that's when I realized I was totally messing up, and I was handling this all wrong. I was telling her everything I advise other people not to do. I was dismissing her feelings by telling her she was fine when she didn't feel fine. I switched gears. "You're right, honey. It looks really, really painful."

She stopped crying and sniffled, nodding.

What did I do wrong at first? Take a moment to imagine this from my daughter's point of view. She hurts herself, but Mom says it's not that bad. My daughter tries again, saying that it is indeed that bad. Then Mom tells her it could have been worse. In other words, I completely dismissed her feelings. Of course, I wasn't trying to do so. I was trying to make her feel better. But despite my good intentions, I discounted my daughter's reality.

Had I not corrected myself, and acknowledged her pain, the message would have been different. It would have been that she could not trust herself to know what hurts her, and she would learn to dismiss what she felt. Now extend that experience of dismissing physical pain to dismissing emotional pain. When you don't learn to take care of your emotions, you learn not to process them; you learn to dismiss them instead of feeling them.

Imagine you're in emotional pain. You're hurting, you're sad, you're upset, and you're worried or anxious. Maybe you say to yourself:

- *Look on the bright side. This really isn't so bad.*
- *People in Africa would love to have such problems.*
- *Things could be worse.*
- *At least you have a roof over your head.*
- *At least you have a job to complain about.*
- *So-and-so didn't really mean to hurt my feelings.*

You may think you're being supportive of yourself or giving yourself a realistic perspective. Nope. This is just a form of dismissing your feelings. Maybe you often say one of the following:

- *I shouldn't feel this way.*
- *What's wrong with me for feeling this way?*
- *Why can't I get a grip?*
- *This is ridiculous.*
- *I hate myself for feeling like this.*

If that's the message you're giving yourself, guess what? You're dismissing your feelings. You're trying to talk yourself out of what you feel instead of allowing yourself to acknowledge and validate what's going on inside. What's a better way to respond? Try something along the lines of this:

- *I'm upset right now because this is an upsetting situation.*
- *Of course I'm angry right now. Who wouldn't be in my situation?*
- *I'm anxious right now, but I won't always feel this way.*

You can survive your feelings. You will feel better in time. When you know that your feelings are simply temporary responses to situations, when you're confident that you can bear whatever it is that feels uncomfortable, you won't eat for comfort or distraction.

The experiences we have as children have a huge impact on how we relate to ourselves and to the world. We learn to treat ourselves based on how we were parented as children. If your parents or caregivers responded to you with anxiety, dismissal, or anger, chances are that you internalized those responses. If a painful or upsetting feeling starts to rise up, you may feel anxious and attempt to stop the anxiety. Consciously or unconsciously a part of you says, "Don't feel, don't feel!" You might tell yourself that it's no big deal and try to push aside the feeling. Or you might get mad at yourself for being upset. If the feeling doesn't stop (and it usually doesn't), you just might find yourself eating for distraction or comfort. As you can see, the past doesn't stay in the past. Unless you heal the wounds of the past, those old dynamics will constantly be repeated in the present. The good news is that just as you learned these dismissive ways of relating to yourself, you can unlearn them and learn new supportive and compassionate ways of relating to yourself. And when you do, you will have lasting change.

REPEATING THE PAST AT WORK

In her second year of college, Toni took a philosophy class with a difficult professor, an older man known to favor some students over others. The professor was dismissive and even contemptuous toward Toni, but she was determined to win him over. She often returned home from class and ordered pizza, eating the whole pie throughout the evening. As she ate slices of pizza, her mind floated to the professor.

"I feel as if there's something I can get from him," Toni said. "I feel it in my bones. I know there's something he can give me, if I can just stick with it."

To understand Toni's hope to win over the professor, we must return to her childhood. When she was growing up, her father openly favored her older brother. Toni could never win over her father. Now, without even realizing it, she was experiencing the professor as a do-over of her childhood. Toni was hoping to win her father's approval through her interaction with her professor, who was essentially a stand-in for her father. Eating pizza was a way of filling the void inside since she never felt she had her father's approval.

In our unconscious, authority figures often represent parents. That's why we sometimes respond to our bosses the same way we responded to our parents, or we expect bosses, teachers, or policemen to treat us the way we were treated as children. Similarly, we can sometimes experience our coworkers like siblings. Rivalries at work are often rooted in tensions from the past. If you had to compete for attention growing up, vying for attention from a boss or not allowing a coworker to get the better of you can be understood as a repetition of your childhood.

When painful or upsetting relationships from the past aren't healed, those relationships play out again in the present. We seek out similar people in an attempt to heal that original relationship. If you had a critical father or mother, and could never win his or her praise or approval, you may be drawn to critical partners, hoping to earn their approval. The problem is that critical people rarely give their approval. Instead the past is replayed instead of allayed. The original family drama is repeated, with different people playing the same roles. The first step to change is to recognize these painful and destructive patterns instead of using food as a comfort or distraction.

BLAME VERSUS EXPLAIN

If you have a hard time thinking about how your past has influenced your present, you're not alone. Lots of people resist the idea that something from the past is affecting their current situation. One example is Stan, who shifted awkwardly in his seat every time we talked about his childhood.

"My parents weren't bad people," he said. "I feel guilty talking about them. I feel bad even getting upset with them."

When Stan was a young child, he played kickball in the streets and often got banged up. He recalled showing his mother a particularly nasty scrape. She said, "You're fine. Stop complaining and go back outside."

Stan grew up to respond to his emotional pain the same way his mother responded to his physical injuries. When his feelings were hurt or he was upset, he told himself, "You're fine. Stop complaining."

Stan never complained. Instead he turned to food, stuffing down his feelings.

By the time he came to see me, Stan tipped the scales at nearly four hundred pounds. He could not walk without getting out of breath. His knees and joints were in constant pain. His blood pressure was sky-high.

Stan had internalized his mother's relationship with his pain. When I pointed this out, he said, "I don't want to blame my mother for my weight. It's not her fault I eat. It's not like she holds a gun to my head."

I told Stan that there is a difference between blaming and explaining. *Blaming* is taking a victim stance, pointing to what happened to you as the reason you're the way you are. *Explaining,* on the other hand, is in the service of understanding and change. Recognizing the relationship between the childhood experiences and his current circumstances is a way of saying, "I understand what happened, and I'm trying to do things differently now."

Stan got better at responding to his hurt or upset feelings. The more he was able to express himself without thinking he was complaining or whining, the less often he ate for distraction. Like Stan's parents, most parents try to do their best. Yet they may respond to their children in ways that are problematic, ranging from somewhat hurtful to downright abusive. When children identify with their parents, the external relationship between parent and child becomes an internalized one, a relationship between different parts of themselves. Children grow up to be adults who treat themselves as they were treated, responding to themselves as their parents once responded to them. When we heal the past, we change the present.

HUNGRY FOR LOVE

Since food is experienced on some level as representing nurturing and love, then recognizing your relationship style, or attachment style, will help you understand your complicated relationship to food. As a reminder, the four basic relationship styles in adults are: anxious-preoccupied, dismissive avoidant, fearful-avoidant, and secure. Each one of them has specific implications when it comes to food. Let's take a closer look.

"Out of Sight, Out of Mind" (Anxious-Preoccupied Relationship Style)

Deidre had been in a relationship for eight years. Her boyfriend loved her, was affectionate and committed, yet Deidre was always waiting for the rug to be pulled out from underneath her. She believed it was just a matter of time before something happened to make her boyfriend change his mind about the relationship and dump her. The fear persisted despite her boyfriend's reassurances that he loved her and wanted to grow old together. Deidre was afraid that marriage would be a "set up" and backfire. The way she saw it, "The higher I climb in life, the farther I'll fall."

Where did this idea come from? Deidre grew up in Australia and enjoyed a perfect and idyllic childhood. She recalled surfing every day, hanging out with friends, playing volleyball on the beach, and feeling as if life was safe, perfect, and beautiful. Deidre felt as if she were living in paradise. Then came the day her parents announced that they were divorcing. Deidre was unprepared for this news and felt as if her world had cracked apart. She was devastated.

As a result of this early experience, Deidre grew up expecting every relationship to end suddenly. She could not allow himself to trust that her boyfriend was there for keeps. The only thing that lessened her anxiety and calmed her down was fast food. Whenever she went through a drive-through, she would have a few minutes of peace in which she was not worrying about having her world turned upside down.

Similarly, Lynette experienced constant anxiety about losing her husband. She and her husband Bill had been together for decades, raised four children, and were madly in love. Yet on a daily basis, Lynette imagined horrible scenarios, thinking about all the possible ways that Bill could be taken from her. In her mind's eye she saw a semi-truck hitting his car on the freeway. She worried that the elevator in his building would break and he would plunge 20 floors to his death. She feared that he would be in the bank at the time of a robbery and get shot. These thoughts were so overwhelming that the only thing that calmed her down was eating until she was in a self-described "food coma."

When Lynette was a child, her father was killed in the Vietnam War. We explored the themes of violence and sudden death that haunted her. For the first time she recognized how the loss of her father influenced her fears about losing Bill. She saw the connection between the experience of loss in the past and the expectation of loss in the future.

Both Deidre and Lynette had experienced trauma related to their attachments. They developed a "Stay close, because if I let you go, you'll leave me" view of connection. People with this attachment style find it difficult to trust in the reliability and availability of those they love or care about. They don't like separation and are afraid that "out of sight" leads to "out of mind." They often seek reassurance that their partner is still there for them.

If this sounds familiar, you may fear that if you allow yourself to connect, you'll eventually lose that love. Even if you're in a relationship, you might feel as if you can never get enough of your boyfriend, girlfriend, husband, wife, or significant other. Even though you have a loved one, you feel a constant fear of losing that love. You may worry that you're "too much" for the other person or worry that he or she will pull away or leave you. If that's the case, you might be in a state of constant anxiety about your relationship. You may be hungry for love but turn to food instead.

We all have wounds from the past that continue to hurt us in the present. When you heal those original wounds by first recognizing they exist and then working through them, everything changes— your relationship to food, to people, and to yourself. Deidre and Lynette explored their fears about trust and mistrust in relationships, recognizing that their fears about relationships were echoes from past emotional pain that had not healed. When they put closure on the past, they both stopped using food for comfort and distraction.

"I Don't Need Anyone" (Dismissive-Avoidant Relationship Style)

Rita owned an online business and worked from home. She conducted most of her business over the Internet, so she rarely interacted personally with other people. And that was just fine with her. She was a proud mommy to three "fur babies" and declared that her dogs were all the company she needed. Rita's only human interaction consisted of the occasional small talk with dog owners at the local dog park. Each night after work she ordered from a local restaurant. Her favorite treat was deep-dish pizza. She ate until she was too stuffed to move, recriminating herself for having no control and feeling despondent and hopeless about ever losing weight.

Applying the Food-Mood Formula, we know that pizza falls into the bulky category and is associated with filling an inner void. By eating pizza until she was stuffed, Rita was filling an emptiness that she consciously denied but unconsciously experienced. When she and I began to delve into her anxieties about relationships, we discovered that she feared losing herself in a relationship. She imagined that she would have to give up her own needs, wishes, likes, and dislikes to make the other person happy. She shuddered as she described the life her mother had given up to be married.

"My mother gave up a career as an investigative journalist to marry my dad. He didn't want her traveling all over the world. He wanted her home with him, where he could control her. She's been dependent on my father ever since and she never had a life of her own."

The possibility that Rita might follow in her mother's footsteps was such a repellant idea that she didn't allow herself any meaningful connection. This kind of attachment style can be understood as "I don't need to be close, I don't want to be close, and I'm keeping my distance." Dismissive-avoidant people are often uncomfortable with closeness. They prize independence, telling themselves and others that they don't need anyone else to be happy.

Underlying this outward disinterest in relationships can be a fear that intimacy will lead to rejection, pain, or loss of self. On some level, the belief is that "if you don't get too close, you won't get hurt." If you turn away from people as a way to protect yourself from potential pain, you may be left feeling too disconnected or lonely, which leaves you vulnerable to using food to fill the void.

By challenging the notion that closeness inevitably leads to loss of independence or selfhood, Rita took baby steps toward connection. As of the writing of this book, she reports that the more she hangs out with people in a way that feels comfortable to her, allowing some connection without feeling smothered by others, the less pizza she is consuming.

"He Went from Hot to Not" (Fearful-Avoidant Relationship Style)

Shelby was only attracted to bad boys. In the first six months that we worked together, she became infatuated with a married man at work, pursued another guy who only dated brunettes (she was blonde), and dated a man who lived in the United Arab Emirates and traveled sporadically to Southern California, where Shelby lived. Whenever a man expressed interest in her, she proclaimed "He's boring!" and never saw him again. Then she met a guy who appeared lukewarm and not that into her, which lit a fire under Shelby. She did everything she could to make him like her. She essentially became the person he was looking for, so he naturally responded by being a lot more interested in her than he was initially. After several months of dating, he suggested that they become exclusive.

Shelby broke up with him a week later. When I asked her what happened, she said, "As soon as he wanted a more permanent thing, it's like he went from hot to not."

Fearful-avoidant adults are in a bind: They simultaneously wish for closeness, yet they also fear intimacy. They often fall in love with someone who's already in a relationship with someone else, or someone who lives too far away to see on a regular basis. They choose partners who are workaholics or have hobbies that take up a lot of time, so they don't have time for the relationship. They are comfortable with the idea of love but terrified of what will happen if they allow themselves to truly bond and connect with another person. They frequently yearn for someone who is unavailable and ardently pursue him or her. If the object of their affection returns their feelings, they generally lose interest, finding distance safer—until the pattern repeats.

There are many reasons for this relationship style. Some people pursue others, only to distance themselves, because they're addicted to the chase and enjoy the experience of pursuit. They don't want an actual relationship because that is threatening on some level. In Shelby's case, we came to understand that on a very deep level she didn't feel deserving of love, and that if she allowed anyone to get close, she would be found out and rejected. By avoiding emotional intimacy, she avoided the pain of expected rejection. Yet at the same time, Shelby was lonely, because she felt the lack of a special relationship. Whenever she felt the acute pain of emptiness and detachment, she binged to the point that she was stuffed. Instead of feeling fulfilled in her relationships, Shelby filled up on food.

Bingeing is a symbolic way to fill up on food as a replacement for love. Shelby faced her fears about intimacy and started seeing relationships as satisfying instead of scary. The more she found satisfaction in connection with others, the less she ate for satisfaction. Like Shelby, when you process your fears about closeness, you can start to enjoy your friendships and connections on a whole new level. Shelby is currently seeing someone new, and although she sometimes feels "squirmy," she's allowing herself to take in the closeness. I feel hopeful that things will shift for her and that one day she can enjoy the richness and depth of love.

"Of Course You Love Me" (Secure Relationship Style)

What does it feel like to have a secure sense of lovability? Consider this: Thousands of actors and actresses come to Hollywood from all over the world, hoping to break into movies and TV. Auditioning can be nerve-wracking, since most of the time they get rejected. In fact, it's estimated that working actors can go on 20 auditions or more for every job they land. That means their booking ratio, as it's called, is 20:1, which is considered a normal booking ratio for someone who earns a living as an actor. Yet, I know an actor who books nearly every part he auditions for. His booking ratio is something like 2:1. By his own admission he isn't any more talented than other actors, so how does he do it?

For one thing, he isn't at all worried about the audition process, which in itself is a rare attitude. Every time an actor enters the casting room, it's an opportunity to get the job. It's also an opportunity to be judged and rejected. Many actors lose out on jobs because they get so nervous.

Not my actor friend Tommy. As he says, "I know the casting directors will love me. Why wouldn't they?" He goes into every audition expecting to be well received by the casting directors. As a result he is always relaxed and comfortable at his auditions. By his own admission, that sense of ease has a lot to do with why he books all these jobs.

Where does this expectation of acceptance come from? Tommy comes from a very supportive family. They make him feel loved and—this is important—lovable. When you feel lovable, you expect that others will like you and love you. That's why it's so easy for him to go into a casting office with positive expectations. It's no surprise that he also had an easy time dating, stayed friends with all his ex-girlfriends, and has a close, loving marriage.

Securely attached people are comfortable with intimacy. They tend to have positive views of themselves and others, and they trust that closeness with another person can be a warm, positive, and mutually satisfying experience. Because they feel satisfied in this area of their lives, they don't use food as a substitute for love.

Cultivating and enjoying fulfilling relationships with other people (as well as with yourself) makes the world an easier, more comfortable place to be. By connecting to others in a meaningful way, you'll find yourself enjoying life and focused more on people instead of your body.

THE FOOD OF LOVE VERSUS THE LOVE OF FOOD

There's a joke from the 1940s in which one man asks another, "Can you tell me what it is that most of us eat at one time or another, yet it's the worst thing in the world for us?"

The second man retorts, "Wedding cake!"

Another phrase comes from the writer George Bernard Shaw, who observed, "There is no love sincerer than the love of food."

Well, there you have it. Marriage is dangerous. Food is trustworthy. If you're focusing on *something* (such as food, weight, body image, and appearance) rather than *someone*, then whatever is going on with food may reflect your conflicts about closeness, intimacy, and trust. Sometimes the "food of love" can be replaced with the "love of food."

I once posted a photo on Facebook that said "I love food" (I "heart" food, actually) and asked people to respond with their first thoughts. What they wrote fell into three different categories:

1. *Those who love food*
2. *Those who have a love-hate relationship with food*
3. *Those who hate-fear food*

Let's start with the first category: Love.

Many people responded that they loved food. They described themselves as foodies and declared that it's good to love food. Several of them pointed out that food is a part of our heritage, of our cultural celebrations, and of our social interactions, and it's essential to our lives. All true.

If you love food, then you probably think food should be enjoyed. And you're right. Food isn't just a source of nourishment; it's one of the pleasures of life. But what if the "love of food" has taken the place of the "food of love?" If you turn to eating instead of connecting with people, if you fill up on food at the expense of having fulfilling relationships, then you're also depriving yourself of the experience of loving and of being loved.

Maybe there's no one in your life and you're eating to symbolically fill the emptiness and the loneliness. Even if you're in a relationship and have a partner, spouse, or family, you might find food easier than people. Lots of people have meals with their husbands, wives, partners, or families and then wait for everyone to go to bed so that they can go into the kitchen and eat. But why?

Sometimes eating is a way of avoiding emotions. Sometimes it's a way of expressing emotions. And sometimes it has to do with not fully trusting relationships.

Maybe it's hard to trust that the person you love or care about will be consistently available. Maybe you don't like separation and you're worried that "out of sight" leads to "out of mind." You binge because you're "hungry" for love, but you don't *trust* love. It could be you're worried you'll never get enough or be satisfied in a relationship.

Let's face it: It can be easier to love food than to trust people. People can be unpredictable and unreliable. They can lie to you, cheat on you, disappoint you, annoy you, and they can change. Unlike people, food is always the same—and always available. If you feel safer with food than with people, you might want to explore your anxieties or expectations about relationships. When you can trust the connection, vulnerability, and closeness of a relationship, you'll be far less likely to use food as a substitute for people.

The second category is the *love-hate* relationship with food. John Bukenas, host of the *Let's Reverse Obesity* podcast, is open about his own love-hate relationship with food. John sometimes loved eating for comfort, but he also told me, "What I hate about food is the control I give it. At times I try to fill up an emptiness, but no matter how much I eat, the emptiness never really goes away."

If you can relate to John, maybe you're overeating because you're lonely. It's a temporary solution, because food in your stomach doesn't actually fill the emptiness in your heart. As I discussed earlier, it's not a substitute for love and connection.

But that's the "love" part of the love-hate relationship. Now let's talk about the "hate":

John went on to say that he and food are in a "knockdown, drag-out fight for control." He said, "Lately I have won more battles than I have lost, but my opponent is cunning and strong. I can never let my guard down."

Notice the way John talks about his battle with food. He sees the part of him that uses food to cope as a separate entity, an enemy with whom he has to do battle. It's hard when the very thing you're trying to control is actually controlling you. If you have a love-hate relationship with food, ask yourself what else in your life you're conflicted about, what other areas feel like a battleground. If you weren't trying to control food, what would you be trying to control? Or are there areas in your life that you are unable to control?

What would you be battling? Or whom?

It can be easier to focus on food or your weight than to deal with an unpredictable boss, teacher, significant other, or friend. You can't control a person, but you can try to control food, turning a relational issue between yourself and someone else into a conflict between yourself and food. Or maybe there is an area in your life that you cannot seem to control, such as your fertility or watching someone you love suffer from an illness. Those feelings of helplessness can also manifest as a desire to control food since you feel powerless to control the situation. When your life feels chaotic, you may focus on controlling food or your weight as a way of managing that painful, difficult state.

Controlling food is also a way of protecting yourself from vulnerability. That's challenging for many people—especially for guys, who are taught to be tough. Men receive the message that they need to man up and be strong. Trying to control food feels active and is a solution to the passivity of vulnerability. Whatever conflicts you may be avoiding by remaining so focused on food and weight don't disappear until you deal with them directly. When you do that, you'll stop distracting yourself with dieting.

The last category is *hate-fear*: Do you ever find yourself just shoving food in your mouth, not even caring what it is, feeling desperate and frenzied? You may eat whatever is in sight, even food you don't like, or uncooked food, or concoctions of protein powder and whatever is in the fridge.

Getting in that binge zone distracts from thoughts you don't want to think and feelings you don't want to feel. Are you afraid of being judged? Do you often avoid social events, fearing there will be no "safe" food, worrying that you either won't be able to control yourself around food or that you'll be judged for how you look?

Whatever your relationship with food—love, love-hate, or hate-fear—remaining invested in weight and body image issues keeps you from having or fully enjoying authentic relationships. It is possible to change your relationship with food and to construct a new way of relating to other people. Ultimately, the goal is to have a positive view of yourself and others and trust that closeness with another person can be a warm, positive, and mutually satisfying experience. When you have that, and can have satisfying mutual relationships, you're less likely to turn to food as a substitute for love and connection and more likely to turn to people.

How do you accomplish that? You start relating to yourself as you want to be treated, or as you treat your friends, and make yourself a priority. When I make this point, the most common reaction I get is something along the lines of "Make myself a priority? I can't do that. It's selfish."

If that resonates with you, it's important to distinguish between being selfish and practicing self-care.

WHAT IS SELF-CARE, ANYWAY?

Recently Lily went on a cruise to Mexico with a group of girlfriends. She proudly reported that none of her friends found out about her lifelong dread of water and ocean liners.

"I was petrified the whole time. All I could think of was *The Poseidon Adventure*," she said. "But they never knew it."

"Why didn't you tell them you're afraid of water?" I asked.

"That would have been selfish," Lily said. "They were so excited about all of us taking a cruise together. I didn't want to spoil it for them."

The definition of "selfish" is having no consideration for other people and being solely concerned with your own interests, or what brings you pleasure or benefits you.

In contrast, the definition of "selfless" is to be more concerned with the needs and wishes of others than with your own. It's the opposite of selfish. It's a problem when these seem like the only two options. If you're not completely selfless, if you have some basic concern about your own well-being, you might feel selfish.

The good news is there's a middle ground: self-care. That means balancing your needs with those of others. Everyone who has flown a commercial airline knows that flight attendants tell passengers, "Parents, if you're traveling with your children and the oxygen masks drop, place a mask over yourself *first*, before attending to your children." If you give away your oxygen, you're of no use to others (and you're likely to suffocate). This can be understood as a metaphor about self-care. If you do not take care of yourself, you're of no use to anyone.

Or, to phrase it another way, "an empty vessel cannot serve."

If you say yes to cake, yes to pizza, yes to chocolate, then maybe you need to start saying no. Not to food but to people. In certain situations saying no to others is like saying yes to yourself. And when you do that, you're far less likely to stuff down your feelings, literally and figuratively.

When my husband and I were dating, we went to the movies a lot. One occasion sticks in my mind. I actually don't remember what movie we saw that night, but I vividly recall the couple in front of us at the ticket line. At first I couldn't tell if they were on their first date or if they had been married forever.

He said, "What do you want to see?"

She said, "Oh, it doesn't matter."

He indicated a poster for a scary horror movie. "What about that one?"

She had that look on her face—you know that look, the one that says, "I so do *not* want to see that movie." Instead she said, "Great, whatever. I'm just happy to be away from the kids for a night."

Okay, so probably not a first date.

The guy said, "Might be gory. I know you don't like blood."

"I'm totally fine with it. Whatever you want is good with me."

It seemed obvious to me that this woman would probably choose sitting in a dentist's chair and getting a root canal to watching that particular movie. Yet she agreed to see it. Why couldn't she say no?

It's not just women who have a hard time saying no or setting limits. One of my guy friends can't say no to anything his boss asks. Stay late? Work over the weekend? Take on an extra project? Reschedule his vacation? He says yes to every request.

Here are some possible and common reasons it might be difficult for you to say no to other people:

- *Feeling guilty—as if it's wrong to choose yourself*
- *Feeling greedy—as if it's greedy to want what you want if someone else wants something different (so they're not greedy if they get what they want, but you are)*
- *Not wanting to come off as difficult—as if saying no makes you difficult and cranky and too much trouble*
- *Not wanting want to upset anyone—as if you're responsible for the feelings of others*
- *Afraid to hurt someone's feelings—as if what the other person wants, thinks, or feels is more important than what you want, think, or feel*
- *Fear of rejection—as if people won't like you or want to be your friend if you disappoint them*
- *Fear of retaliation—as if saying no may have terrible consequences. (My friend thought if he said no to working over the weekend, he wouldn't get promoted.)*

How does this relate to bingeing or overeating? Well, if you give up what you want to make other people happy, which is sometimes called "people pleasing," then you're likely carrying around some resentment or anxiety. Instead of recognizing that you feel upset, you may use food for distraction because while you're eating you're not thinking about what's bothering or upsetting you.

You may even turn that resentment or anxiety onto yourself. Instead of feeling upset that you didn't set limits or didn't speak up about what you really wanted or needed, you get upset because you ate too much, or too much of the wrong thing, or because you weigh more than you think you should. You feel anxious or guilty about how much weight you might gain instead of feeling anxiety about your friendship or your bonds with other people. Eating and then focusing on weight and body image is a distraction from and a displacement of these feelings of anxiety, resentment, and guilt.

What's the answer? Say no to others and say yes to yourself. That can be tough, especially when on some level you think that what you need, want, or feel doesn't matter as much as the needs, wants, and feelings of others. Maybe you believe that you don't have the right to set boundaries that protect yourself.

Challenge the idea that it's selfish to set limits. Let's review the definitions again: Being "selfish" means having no consideration for other people and only being concerned with your own interests or well-being. Being "selfless" means being more concerned with the needs and wishes of others than with your own, which leaves you empty, deprived, angry, and lonely. Between selfishness and selflessness is self-*care,* balancing your needs with those of others, giving yourself permission to have needs and wants that are just as important as those of other people.

If your default is to be selfless, saying yes to people when you really want to say no, consider how you learned to make other people's needs or wants more important than yours. We all grow up with different messages about self-sacrifice. Some people consider it noble. The message is that it's noble to give up your desires or needs to make someone else happy. You may even feel like a good person for denying yourself. Occasionally it's necessary to think about others, but if you're always giving up your wishes to take care of those of others, then it's harmful to you.

Nearly all of our values and ideas about the world come from the past. The messages you received in childhood about asserting your rights and expressing your emotions influence the way you operate in the world today. One of my patients, Katrina, came to America from Eastern Europe as a child and was teased by other children. They made fun of her accent, mocked her difficulty with English, and jeered at the food her mother packed for lunch. When Katrina told her parents that she felt sad and lonely, they told her to ignore the taunts. They always asked if she had done anything to cause the other kids to make fun of her. The message was that she should ignore bad treatment and also focus on the other person rather than on herself. Katrina found herself turning to food for comfort and solace.

It's no surprise that Katrina grew up tolerating poor treatment from others. Her friends often took advantage of her. Most of the guys she dated were self-absorbed and inconsiderate. Her latest boyfriend never went to Katrina's house because it was too far, yet he expected her to drive to see him every weekend. Katrina felt guilty for resenting this and often ate to escape the guilt.

> "Self-sacrifice doesn't make you a better person. It makes you a deprived person."

Self-sacrifice doesn't make you a better person. It makes you a deprived person. If you don't consistently meet your needs and wants, you're likely to transfer those needs to food. Maybe you comfort yourself with something sweet or express your anger with crunchy food. Maybe you eat so much it hurts, converting emotional pain into physical pain. The answer is to empower yourself to balance your needs with those of others. In many cases, when you say no to others, you're saying yes to yourself. If you're in a situation where you're afraid to speak up or say no, here are some guidelines for how to handle it:

- *Don't apologize, don't make excuses, don't justify or explain. Do offer other options, if the situation calls for it. Let's start with the people at the movie. The wife could have said, "You're right, horror movies aren't my favorite. Let's pick something we both want to see." My friend could tell his boss, "I can't reschedule my weekend, but I'm willing to stay late once or twice during the week." (In other words, compromise.)*

- *If someone asks you to babysit her kids and you don't want to do it, you can say, "No, I'm not going to be able to do that, but would you like me to look at profiles on Care.com?"*

- *If a friend asks to borrow money, you can say, "I under-stand you're in a tough place right now, but I make it a rule not to lend money to friends." That way it's not personal— you're not denying your friend in particular. This is your rule; these are your boundaries.*

- *If someone pushes it, if he pleads, telling you he's in a bind, what is he going to do, please, please, please, just this once, acknowledge that he's in a tough place, and then repeat that it just doesn't work for you. "I know you're in a bind, but that just doesn't work for me." Acknowledge his need by saying something like, "I know you really need childcare or money . . . " And then set the limit: "But that's not going to work for me."*

If you're afraid of hurting people's feelings or making them mad, that's a sign that you're not valuing your time, your money, your likes and dislikes. When you devalue yourself it feels bad, and when you feel bad, you're more likely to eat for comfort and distraction. Many of us are good at meeting the needs of others while totally ignoring our own needs. When you're taught that self-sacrifice is noble, you cannot differentiate between being selfish and practic-ing self-care. Consistently practicing self-care helps you meet your needs so you won't use food for comfort or distraction. This may be challenging at first, but practice makes progress. In time, setting boundaries will be second nature!

JUST SAY NO

Think about two recent occasions when you said yes to someone else's request when you really wanted to say no. Here's your chance to rewrite that conversation so the next time something similar happens, you will know how to respond.

❈ ❈ ❈

You now know that the way you cope with your feelings may be rooted in your past. Many of your behaviors were likely learned from a parental figure or some other relative or authority figure who taught you—whether consciously or unconsciously—not to express your emotions. But when you hide or repress your emotions and isolate yourself from others, you miss out on the kind of fulfilling intimacy that food will never provide. Food is always a temporary Band-Aid at best because those emotions will continue to surface. Validate your emotional pain instead of dismissing it and you will no longer need to eat for comfort or distraction. Practicing self-care and saying no to others and yes to yourself can empower you to value yourself.

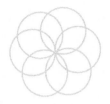

CHAPTER 5

Win the Internal Tug-of-War

Yphou know that feeling when you rationally know something to be true, yet the feeling doesn't match up with what you logically know and believe? That's because it's not logical— it's psychological. We try to resolve that internal tug-of-war in various ways, including by distracting ourselves from discomfort by focusing on our diets, counting calories or fat grams, and being preoccupied with our weight.

> "That's because it's not logical—it's psychological."

What you weigh becomes less of a problem when you focus on what's weighing on you. That's why we're going to explore the various ways we deny, deflect, repress, or otherwise push away uncomfortable thoughts, feelings, and conflicts. These are often called defense mechanisms, but I like to think of them as ways of protecting us from pain that also ultimately hurt us. They include mind reading, turning on the self, intellectualizing, minimizing, bargaining, slave driving, and overdoing. Do you ever assume that someone else is thinking that you are fat or judging you for what you are eating? Or do you apologize profusely when you are late but never express anger when someone else is? Do you minimize your problems the moment you begin to express some serious emotions? I will help you to understand what's really happening below the surface. Once you begin to recognize these behaviors, you can more easily let go of them and address the underlying emotions that are causing you to turn to food for comfort.

YOU PROBABLY THINK . . . (MIND READING)

When you walk into a room filled with strangers, what are your initial thoughts? Do you imagine the best possible scenario? Do you think, *These people are interested in me and can't wait to meet me?* Or do you think the worst? *These people think I'm fat . . . boring . . . stupid . . . and they don't want to have anything to do with me. They can see that there's something about me that's different or somehow unlikable.*

I'm going to take a wild guess and presume you do not work for a psychic network. Therefore, you do not actually know what's in another person's mind. Many of us feel as if the world is scrutinizing us and finding us wanting. Believing that other people are thinking the worst can also be subtle. Consider the following examples:

Arturo sat on the couch in my office, telling me about his weekend. He'd seen a movie and spent time with his girlfriend, and he also played golf all day on Sunday. I listened without interruption or comment. I didn't speak. I didn't say a single word.

He looked at me and nodded. "You're right, I should have done some work this weekend. I can't believe how lazy I am."

On another occasion, Corinne wept in frustration as she described a recent problem at work. She blew her nose and grabbed tissues from the box, taking the last of them. She shook her head apologetically. "You probably think I'm such a crybaby."

More recently my friend Kellie and I had dinner, and at the end of the meal, she ordered dessert. After giving the server an order for apple pie a la mode, Kellie gave me a sheepish look. "I know what you're thinking," she said. "I have no business eating apple pie."

I didn't think Arturo was lazy. I didn't think Corinne was a crybaby. I didn't think that Kellie had no business ordering dessert. Arturo, Corinne, and Kellie were projecting the critical thoughts they had about themselves onto me and then believing that I was thinking the same thoughts. So where did those critical perceptions come from? They came from the usual place: the past. Arturo's father always accused him of being a slacker, and he had internalized that view of himself. He thought I was viewing him through his father's eyes. Corinne grew up in a family that didn't tolerate emotions or tears, which were viewed as signs of weakness. She imagined that I was viewing her tears contemptuously, as her family members did whenever someone expressed emotion. Kellie's mother constantly monitored her weight, and Kellie thought I was doing so too. She transferred the shaming experience with her mother onto me.

If you think other people are critical, indifferent, exasperated, or angry, you're a lot more likely to use food as a substitute for love and comfort. Conversely, when you trust that others like you and think the best of you, you feel good. When you feel good, there's no need to distract yourself with food.

IT'S NOT YOU, IT'S ME
(TURNING ON THE SELF)

Sloane arrived twenty minutes late to her session, looking flustered. "I'm so sorry," she apologized. "It's rude and disrespectful for me to be this late."

She explained that her toilet had overflowed and the plumber had a flat tire on the way to her house. He was late and took longer than expected to make the repair, which in turn made Sloane late for her appointment.

"You must be so upset with me," she said.

"Why would I be upset?" I asked.

"Because I was late," she said, as if this was quite obvious.

I wondered if she thought the plumber had been rude and disrespectful. Was she upset with him the way she imagined that I would be upset with her?

"Not at all," she said. "It wasn't his fault that he had a flat tire. I don't have the right to be upset."

"What do you mean, the 'right' to be upset?" I asked.

"I can't be mad if there's a good reason for what happened."

Sloane believed that if she could explain a situation logically, she wasn't allowed to have any feelings about it. Yet, although she expected me to be upset at her for being late, for circumstances outside her control, she couldn't give herself the same right.

"You know what does upset me?" Sloane added. "The bagel and cream cheese I ate for breakfast. That was such a bad choice. I should have had an English muffin and jelly. I'm always making the wrong choices when it comes to food. I'm never going to lose weight."

Sloane continued to criticize her weight, her lack of control, and various other perceived deficiencies. She didn't allow herself to be upset that she'd been kept waiting, whatever the circumstances, and instead expressed her frustration by turning on herself and finding fault with her body and food choices.

This is what is known as "turning on the self." I call it the "boomerang" effect: Instead of directing your feelings outward, toward the people or situations that make you feel a certain way, you turn those feelings on yourself. Instead give yourself permission to feel whatever you feel without judgment or criticism. Think emotional Frisbee, not boomerang. Let those feelings fly out and they won't return to you.

WHAT'S THE POINT OF FEELING YOUR EMOTIONS? (INTELLECTUALIZING)

Yasmine had a horrible boss. Worse than Meryl Streep's character in *The Devil Wears Prada*, who was scornful, insulting, dismissive, mean, and unreasonable. She was a dream boss compared to Yasmine's employer, who often told her she could not do anything right. He criticized her performance. He gave specific instructions on what to do, and even if she followed them to the letter he'd find mistakes.

One day Yasmine said, "I have a confession to make," and she proceeded to tell me everything she'd eaten since our last session. She was upset with herself and disgusted with her weight. She accused herself of being a failure, believing she couldn't do anything right.

I suggested that she was taking the anger she felt toward her boss and turning it on herself. I told her, "The way you talk to yourself affects the way you feel. The way you feel affects the way you eat. So if you're self-critical, you feel terrible, which makes you binge for comfort."

Yasmine said, "So what? How is realizing that supposed to help me? What do I do with that information?"

She was being logical, going into her head as a way of staying out of her feelings. To stop that cycle, Yasmine needed to express her feelings about her boss so she wouldn't direct them at herself.

She looked horrified at the suggestion. "I can't do that. I'd be fired on the spot."

I explained that expressing her feelings didn't mean actually telling her boss what she thought. Instead she needed to process them with me or talk with friends. When she expressed those feelings, she would stop using food to direct her anger inward.

Yasmine had difficulty being angry with her boss but easily turned her anger inward. Bingeing did two things for her: First, it provided comfort and helped her numb her feelings. Second, it gave her a way to express all that bottled-up anger by directing it inward. Instead of saying, "My boss is out of control, and I'm so upset at how I'm being treated because I have no control," she said, "See how out of control I am with food?"

Yasmine was not convinced. "What's the point of talking about my feelings? It won't change anything."

In one sense she was absolutely right. Her boss was not going to change. Like Yasmine, we all have encountered people and situations that we can't change. But we can change how we feel about and respond to those situations. It's likely that at some point in your life you have experienced loss, the death of someone you know or love. When a person dies, do you say, "Well, he's gone or she's gone, and there's nothing I can do about it, so what's the point of crying?"

> "We don't change the situation by allowing ourselves to process our feelings; we change how we feel about the situation."

Of course not. Whether you attend a wake or sit shiva or mourn in some other way, these rituals help you grieve the person you lost. You feel a terrible loss and emptiness. And you eventually start feeling better. The person you lost lives on in your memory and in your thoughts, but the intensity of that loss diminishes. The situation has not changed, but it doesn't hurt as much. We don't change the situation by allowing ourselves to process our feelings; we change how we feel about the situation.

You might be wondering why Yasmine had such a hard time being upset at her terrible boss. As you can probably guess by now, the answer to a current problem is usually found in the past. That was the case for Yasmine, whose parents worked long hours at their business, so she spent most afternoons with her erratic, unpredictable grandfather. He didn't merely get frustrated or irritated or upset. He got *furious*. He expressed himself by yelling, finger-pointing, name-calling, using sarcasm, and throwing things. Yasmine grew up equating anger with being out of control and scary. She feared that if she got angry that would make her just as bad, as threatening, and as scary as her grandfather. She had no model for expressing anger in an appropriate way.

When we began to talk about how her experience with her grandfather had influenced her ability to express these feelings, Yasmine gave yet another intellectual response. She said in a very matter-of-fact way, "I guess I can see how a person would have resentment toward a grandfather like that. I can see how a person would be affected by that."

Notice how Yasmine talked about "a person would have resentment toward a grandfather like that" instead of how *she* felt having a close relative whose anger terrified her. Yasmine was eventually able to express how she felt about both her grandfather and her boss. She got mad, outraged, incensed, and she let loose with some pretty creative swear words. She released all of her anger, and when she did that she stopped being so hard on herself.

That's when she stopped bingeing.

If you say things like, "What's the point of talking about it? It won't change anything," or "Other people have it so much worse than I do. I have no right to complain," question those ideas. If you talk about how "people" might feel in your situation, rather than how *you* feel, you might be too much in your head and not enough in your heart.

Whether you're trying to think away your anger, like Yasmine, or deal with other feelings such as sadness, helplessness, anxiety, fear, guilt, worry, or shame, those emotions need your attention, not your condemnation. When you think less and feel more, you're less likely to turn to food when you're upset. When you get out of your head, you'll stay out of the fridge.

IT COULD BE WORSE (MINIMIZING)

Talia wept, her shoulders heaving with pain. She'd had a difficult conversation with her father the previous night. She had just been accepted to medical school at a prestigious local university and rushed home to report the news of her achievement to her parents.

Talia had hoped to make her parents proud. Her father had responded by saying, "Too bad you didn't get into Yale."

"Nothing I do is ever good enough," she sobbed. "It will never be enough. *I'll* never be enough."

Then, gathering herself together, she took a deep breath and dabbed at her eyes.

"I don't know what I'm complaining about," she said. "It's not as if something really terrible happened to me. I didn't get raped or attacked. I don't have cancer. In the grand scheme of things, many people have it much worse."

Talia minimized her upset feelings as a way of denying how devastated she was by her father's response. Usually she binged until she was physically in pain as a way of distracting herself from these emotional wounds. If you tell yourself "it's not that bad" or "it could be worse," you're dismissing your feelings. There are two types of wounds: One is a huge, traumatic event, the equivalent of getting stabbed in the heart with a butcher knife. The other type of wound is a repetitive experience of smaller traumas, like a thousand small cuts. Whether your emotional pain involves a specific incident in your life or a pattern of responses that were hurtful, that pain needs your attention, not your condemnation.

Several years ago a deadly tsunami in Japan killed thousands of people and wiped out whole villages. Around the same time, a friend of mine lost everything in a house fire. Decades of family photos and mementos from family vacations went up in smoke. This was a devastating loss, one that was made even more difficult by the reactions of others.

"Look on the bright side. You're lucky to have a house to rebuild," someone told her. "Those people in Japan lost their houses and their lives."

"It could have been worse," said many other people.

"You were lucky nobody got hurt. Things are replaceable," they said.

This kind of comparison creates a false equivalency. If you break your arm snowboarding and your best friend breaks a leg, that doesn't make your broken arm less painful. If your house is flooded and you need to redo all the flooring, and your neighbor's house goes up in flames and burns to the ground, you do not have less of a right to be upset. If you want to lose fifty pounds, and your friend needs to lose one hundred and fifty, you're not expected to be happy that you have less weight to lose.

We can all be thankful we're not in Africa dealing with an AIDs epidemic and with other dire conditions. We are grateful that we do not experience the horror of a tsunami ripping our world apart. We aren't refugees from war or terrorism. What's happening in other parts of the world is tragic, but those situations do not take away our right to be upset about the problems and issues that affect us. When we minimize our feelings, we use food as a coping mechanism.

WHEN I LOSE WEIGHT, I'LL GET HIM BACK (BARGAINING)

Do you think that losing weight will change your life? Many people believe that by changing the number on the scale they can change the way they feel—and the way people respond to them. Francesca thought things were going really well with her boyfriend of a year. When he asked her to come over because he had something important to talk about, she thought he was going to propose.

Instead he broke up with her.

Did she cry? Did she get upset? Yes, but not for long.

Soon she was telling me, "I know how to get him back. I'm going to lose fifteen pounds and look so smoking hot, he'll be so sorry he broke up with me. He'll be begging to get back together."

Francesca wasn't dealing with the pain and loss of the relationship. She wasn't considering how it affected her. She certainly wasn't working through her feelings. Instead she was thinking about getting her boyfriend to come back. In her mind, the way to do that was by changing her appearance.

Lose fifteen pounds and, *voilà*, she'd be irresistible.

Francesca thought she could control her ex-boyfriend by controlling her weight. Like Francesca, lots of people think that when they lose weight, their lives will improve and they'll be more confident, outgoing, relaxed, and happy. They make statements like the following:

- *"When I lose weight, I'll start dating."*
- *"When I lose weight, I'll look for a new job."*
- *"When I lose weight, I'll finally have the courage to leave my spouse."*
- *"When I fit into those jeans in the back of my closet, I'll be happy."*

These are all some form of when/then. *When* the number on the scale is where you want it to be, *then* life will be better. If this resonates with you, you may believe, like Francesca, that by controlling your weight you can manage many aspects of your life, including your likability, lovability, and overall happiness. But you can't control the world by controlling your weight. For Francesca, focusing on losing weight was a way to avoid the pain of the breakup and her powerlessness over the situation.

Feeling powerless is connected to vulnerability and dependency, both of which can be extremely difficult. Two responses to powerlessness are getting angry and getting busy. Anger is an active emotion, whereas powerlessness is a passive emotion. Getting mad keeps you from the vulnerable, raw, painful, or depressing states of helplessness. Being busy is also way of turning passive to active.

Eating, counting calories, focusing on achievements, and going to the gym all the time are all ways of "doing" rather than "feeling."

Francesca eventually talked about some of the issues she and her ex-boyfriend had throughout their relationship. One problem was that he'd been married before and wasn't sure if he wanted more kids, while she definitely wanted kids of her own. She started to question herself and her wishes.

"Maybe I should just be happy being a stepmom. Maybe it's too much to want my own biological kids." Then she paused. "I bet he'd want kids with me if I were thinner."

Notice how she shifted from being worried about wanting too much to thinking about being too much, being too big, weighing too much. This is an example of how our perceptions of ourselves can be influenced by emotions, needs, and wants. If you often feel as if you're too much for others, that you're too demanding, or that you burden people with your needs, the sense of wanting too much, or needing too much, can be unconsciously experienced as seeing yourself as literally too big.

Think about what's "too much" about you and where you got that idea about yourself. People who grow up in families in which emotionality is labeled "dramatic" or "oversensitive" or "ridiculous" learn to dismiss their feelings and often believe that they feel things too intensely and are more sensitive than other people. They feel as if their emotions are too much and imagine that they're too much for others. This can then be expressed in concrete, physical terms about their size. Instead of feeling too much, they "are" too much.

It's one thing to want to lose weight for health reasons, but if you are trying to change your life by changing your weight, take a moment and consider what your weight means symbolically. Weight can represent the qualities you want to get rid of, such as shyness, insecurity, anxiety, and so forth—losing weight becomes equivalent to losing those unacceptable "parts" of yourself. It's easier to focus on losing weight than to think about shedding disappointments, fears, concerns, worries, and anxieties.

Alex was one hundred pounds overweight and insecure about his appearance. Social situations were painful because he felt awkward talking with other people. He imagined that when he lost the weight, he would become more confident and more social and that he'd have more friends. As he incorporated the self-care strategies I taught him, he began to lose weight. Eventually he lost more than one hundred pounds. He felt an overwhelming and liberating sense of confidence. For a while.

Soon new insecurities resurfaced. Alex began to worry that he wasn't smart enough. He didn't know enough about politics or the stock market, and he didn't understand business the way he should. He avoided talking to people at parties because he thought they'd realize he was not as smart as he seemed. Whereas he once worried about the size of his stomach, now Alex was concerned with the size of his intellect.

Losing weight doesn't mean you lose the qualities and characteristics about yourself that you don't like. Losing weight doesn't change you; it only changes the number on the scale or the size on the labels of your jeans. If you have fears or insecurities, when you lose weight those insecurities attach to something else about you. Alex thought losing one hundred pounds would change his life, but what he really needed to lose were his insecurities about himself.

Alex thought his problem with women stemmed from being a homebody. He'd rather stay home and watch a movie than go out to clubs or parties.

I asked, "What's wrong with being a homebody?"

He assumed women preferred guys who rode motorcycles or drove expensive sports cars and took them to fancy restaurants and clubs. I suggested that all women don't like just one kind of man, just as all men don't like just one kind of woman. Together we questioned the idea that being a chill-out-at-home kind of guy made him inferior in some way, or unattractive.

Alex is now married to a woman who also enjoys staying home and watching movies on the couch. Occasionally they go out for a night on the town. His wife isn't interested in fancy sports cars, and she thinks motorcycles are scary, not sexy. When Alex accepted his authenticity and remained true to his values and principles, he found someone who was a good match. Isn't that wonderful? I love a happy ending.

Losing weight is like moving to a different city or a different country, hoping to have a different life. Wherever you go, there you are. When you lose the negative ideas about yourself, you'll be happier and feel good about yourself. That's when you lose weight for good.

WHAT QUALITIES DO YOU WANT TO LOSE?

Forget the realities of the scale for a moment. Consider the "bad" parts of yourself that you want to get rid of, and question what would be different if you lost weight. As much as we want to believe that losing weight will transform us, losing weight doesn't actually change who you are as a person.

Challenge the idea that there's something deficient, unlikable or unlovable about you and that losing weight will solve those problems or fix you. Take a moment and give some thought to what qualities (not physical characteristics) you think you need to get rid of. How did you come to believe those qualities were unacceptable? Is there another way of looking at them?

THE MORE I DO, THE BETTER I AM (SLAVE DRIVING)

Brenda perched on the couch, an open notebook on her lap and a pen poised over the page, holding my gaze. She looked like a schoolgirl ready to take notes.

"I need some tools to deal with my compulsive overeating. I don't want to talk about my family or about the past. I just want you to tell me what to do."

Brenda spent each evening on the computer answering e-mails and doing online research for work, the TV blaring in the background and a crochet project in her lap. As long as she was multitasking, she was fine. Without those distractions she turned to food.

"So," she asked, pen at the ready, "what do I need to do?"

I said, "You need to do less."

Brenda blinked in confusion. "Do less? What is that supposed to mean?"

I explained that her relentless pursuit of accomplishment was likely a distraction from uncomfortable thoughts and emotions. When she could "be" with herself, she would no longer need to do so much—or to eat when she was stressed.

Brenda considered just "being" with herself a waste of time. She had no concept of what it might be like to value herself because of who she is instead of because of her *accomplishments*. Like Brenda, many of us define ourselves by what we do, and we miss out on the richness of simply being. Author and self-development coach Dr. Wayne Dyer once said, "I am a human being, not a human doing. Don't equate your self-worth with how well you do things in life. You aren't what you do. If you are what you do, then when you don't . . . you aren't." Deepak Chopra makes a similar point in a television advertisement for Microsoft, asserting, "I am a PC and a human being. Not a human doing. Not a human thinking. A human being."

Wayne Dyer and Deepak Chopra are in the minority. Our society often values productivity and accomplishment above everything else. If you grow up in a family (and/or a culture) that is primarily or solely interested in what you're achieving, you learn to value yourself by being productive; it becomes the basis of your self-esteem. When other people express interest solely in your accomplishments, you learn to value yourself only for what you have achieved and you may devalue yourself when you are not actively achieving or when you experience failure. When they dismiss or devalue your feelings, you learn to do the same. Feelings become frightening and a source of anxiety, and in the absence of other ways to cope, eating is a way of dealing with all the curveballs that life throws at you.

"Doing" can serve as a distraction from your emotions. It can take the form of working all the time, going to the gym or being online every night, running errands instead of relaxing, having the TV on at all hours, filling every evening with activities, constantly thinking about what you need to accomplish next, making lists, or thinking about fat grams, calories, and the number on the scale.

"Being" puts you in touch with your emotions. It means staying aware of your thoughts and feelings and having the ability to comfort, support, and soothe yourself when you're upset.

If it's difficult for you to relax and you keep yourself busy doing ten things at once, always thinking about your next project, you may use "doing" to escape "feeling." When you're alone and learn to "be" with the thoughts, emotions, and conflicts that arise when you aren't productive, you may be surprised at what surfaces.

This was the case with Ross, a successful businessman who woke up at five o'clock each morning for a grueling five-mile run through his hilly neighborhood and then worked hard during the day, running his corporation. He spent nights entertaining clients at upscale restaurants. His day typically ended at midnight, when he visited his neighborhood supermarket and bought food that he would then binge on when he returned home.

Ross was an attractive, fit man who drove an expensive car, lived alone in a multimillion-dollar estate, and could not understand his late-night binges. He looked bewildered as he talked about them.

"I built my business from nothing. I'm successful. Why can't I beat this thing with food? It's the only problem in my life."

I asked what it felt like to talk about this issue.

Ross shrugged. "I just need some tools to deal with it. I need to figure out how to make it work."

I was struck by the way Ross talked about his conflict with food as if it were a business problem that needed to be solved rather than a painful personal issue.

Ross grew up in a large, poor family, the oldest of six children. His depressed mother often stayed in the bedroom for days or even weeks, leaving Ross to tend to his siblings. His father came home late from work, usually drunk, and spent each evening staring at the television. Affection in the house was as scarce as money. From an early age, Ross recognized that his parents were unable to take adequate care of him and his five siblings. He turned to accomplishment as a way to distract from painful feelings and keep things organized. He knew it was up to him to "make it work."

And work he did. Starting with a paper route at age twelve, he put himself through college, then graduate school. He earned a business degree and achieved millionaire status before age thirty.

Yet Ross was unsatisfied. There was always more to do, more to accomplish. Nothing was ever enough. Relentless productivity was his strategy to build a better life for himself as a child. As an adult, Ross was still trying to outrun his feelings by staying busy all the time.

At night when he was finally alone and there were no distractions, Ross ate until his stomach hurt. The food symbolically filled his internal emptiness and converted painful emotions to physical sensations. Instead of heartache, Ross experienced a stomachache.

As the treatment progressed, Ross identified powerful feelings of loneliness that stemmed from childhood. In the early years of his life he could not rely on others to take care of him, so he idealized self-reliance. He didn't trust people, whom he unconsciously feared would disappoint or criticize him. He could not turn to people for connection or comfort. Instead Ross turned to food. Unlike people, food didn't disappoint. Unlike people, food was consistent and always available.

Through therapy Ross learned to process his ambivalence about relationships and began to form connections with others. As he connected with people, he felt less lonely and more fulfilled. Food was no longer his best friend, and he stopped bingeing.

Laura had a lot in common with Ross. She was always in a hurry and she had tons of energy. (She was also highly caffeinated at all times.) If multitasking were an Olympic skill, she would have been a gold medalist. Relaxation meant putting a movie on TV and sitting on the couch with her laptop open, a cell phone nearby, plus a bunch of magazines and a big bowl of popcorn. She was obsessed with popcorn and was always trying to find some low-calorie equivalent of movie popcorn. While Laura watched a movie, she checked her e-mails; updated her Instagram, Twitter, and Facebook; read magazines; and ate popcorn. She considered this "doing nothing." Then Laura started going out with John, an artist who was into yoga and meditation. She liked John, which is why she was willing to give meditation a try. John lit some candles . . . they settled on pillows . . . closed their eyes . . . and John told Laura to focus on her breath and tell herself, "I am calm, I am relaxed, and I am happy."

Laura closed her eyes and thought, "I am calm. I am relaxed."

Her next thought was "And I am *bored*. This is so boring."

Then she started counting fat grams and calories, adding up what she'd eaten that day. She started thinking about popcorn and the difference between kettle corn and regular popcorn, whether the fiber in popcorn made it an actual diet food or not. Instead of letting go of stress, Laura meditated on popcorn and the calorie-burning possibilities of yoga.

Laura and John continued dating, so she kept meditating. Usually her thoughts were about dieting and losing weight, until one day she allowed her mind to finally relax and wander. That's when she started thinking about her father, who had abandoned the family when Laura was six years old.

Laura hadn't allowed herself to think too much about her dad, and as a result she never really processed that loss. She'd always told herself she was better off without her father, that she didn't even remember him that well, that her stepdad was more like a dad than her real dad, and that everything happens for a reason.

Laura's best memory of her father involved going to a retro movie screening of *Willy Wonka & the Chocolate Factory* and sharing a bag of popcorn. Now, it could be that Laura just happened to like eating popcorn when she watched movies, as lots of people do. Or it was her way of trying to be close to the father she lost. Maybe both.

As a "human doing," Laura stayed busy and kept her mind occupied at all times. By focusing on her weight, she avoided the pain and anger she felt about being abandoned by her father, feelings that had never been felt but that she was carrying around with her.

Only when she stopped focusing on dieting, when she was "being" in the moment, did those feelings become available to her again. She had to heal the past by dealing with it, so that she would not use work and food to avoid her true feelings.

When you're a "human doing," you may focus on accomplishment, productivity, and multitasking as a way of avoiding difficult emotions or conflicts. Also, eating gives you something to *do*, an activity that distracts from uncomfortable states of mind.

Don't get me wrong—I am in favor of being productive. I'm all for it, as long as there's balance. Yet as Socrates once said, "Beware the barrenness of a busy life." I think that means staying busy keeps us from ourselves and prevents us from appreciating connections with people, from enjoying the quieter, more reflective moments of life. It means that if you don't take time to smell those proverbial roses, your life will be empty and meaningless.

Beware the barrenness—the emptiness, the impoverishment—of a busy life. As I mentioned earlier, our society values productivity and accomplishment. If you grow up in an environment that is primarily or solely interested in what you are doing, accomplishing, and achieving, you learn to value yourself by being productive; it becomes the basis of your self-esteem.

If you're a "human doing," the feelings involved in "being" can become a source of anxiety. Bingeing or overeating is a way of coping with those feelings. So is staying busy and focused on achievements. *Doing* can serve as a distraction from your emotions. It can take the form of:

- *Working all the time*
- *Being online all the time*
- *Going to the gym*
- *Running errands constantly*
- *Having the TV on all the time*
- *Going out and seeing friends all the time*
- *Thinking about what you need to do next/making lists*
- *Thinking about calories, fat grams, the number on the scale*
- *Eating*

Being puts you in touch with your emotions. Being is:

- *Being okay with being alone*
- *Staying aware of thoughts and feelings*
- *Comforting and soothing yourself with words*
- *Relaxing*

Remember how Laura thought she was bored? Boredom is about wanting to do something. The way to alleviate boredom is to engage in an activity that may be productive or simply fun. If that doesn't change your mood, or if you often feel unsettled, then maybe you're not really bored. Laura was not actually bored; she was uncomfortable and using boredom to cover up what was going on inside.

> "Boredom is what's called an umbrella emotion, which means that it covers up other feelings such as anxiety, sadness, anger, fear, guilt, and other uncomfortable states."

Boredom is what's called an umbrella emotion, which means that it covers up other feelings such as anxiety, sadness, anger, fear, guilt, and other uncomfortable states. Laura believed that she was bored, but she was actually anxious about being alone with herself, alone with her thoughts, because when her mind was quieter, she was more in touch with painful memories. She was busy all the time as a way of keeping those memories, and the corresponding feelings, at bay, yet she was a slave to business.

The key to change is allowing yourself to be a human being, not a human doing. When you can be with yourself and process any feelings or conflicts you might experience when you're in that place of being, you're less likely to use food as a distraction from what's uncomfortable. If you're sad, you need to cry or express that sadness. If you're mad, you need to express that as well. If you're feeling anxious or guilty or upset, you have to process those emotions.

As I've mentioned before, *when you feel, you will heal.*

You are not what you do. Think about what kind of a human being you are. Are you a loving person? An honest person? Are you kind, generous, a good friend, loyal, understanding, compassionate, honest, helpful?

Ross dealt with his conflicts about depending on other people and started connecting more with others. He stopped bingeing on food as a way of symbolically filling his emptiness. Laura worked through the painful experience of her father's abandonment and rejection and found herself much less interested in staying busy and eating popcorn. Like Ross and Laura, when you allow yourself to experience a range of thoughts and emotions, and connect to other people in a way that feels satisfying, you'll find true liberation from bingeing.

❁ ❁ ❁

Did you find yourself relating to any of the defense mechanisms in this chapter? Do you often project your thoughts about yourself onto others or your anger toward others onto yourself? Do you stay in your head or keep yourself constantly busy in order to avoid your feelings? Or when you do release some of your emotions, do you then immediately minimize them? Are you stuck in a "when/then" scenario, believing that your life will get better when you eventually lose the weight? Once you acknowledge these behaviors, you can finally begin to resolve that tug-of-war that causes you to focus on food or the number on the scale instead of confronting your uncomfortable emotions, and healing can begin. In the next chapter we'll take a look at some of the fears that may be keeping you stuck.

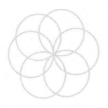

CHAPTER 6

Stop the Sabotage

So far we've explored how feelings, thoughts, and inner conflicts trigger bingeing. You learned several strategies designed to help you shift your relationship with yourself and with others. By making peace with yourself and healing your relationships, you started creating changes with food. That's the good news. The bad news is that once you start losing weight, you may find yourself sabotaging your weight-loss efforts.

A few months into treatment, Dawn discovered that she had lost weight without trying. A week earlier, she weighed herself for the first time in several months and was astonished to find that she had lost seventeen pounds. She was not dieting or going to the gym. The only thing she was doing differently was being nice to herself. The weight loss was a result of recognizing her emotions, processing them, and comforting herself with supportive self-talk instead of turning to food. Initially Dawn was absolutely delighted with the unexpected seventeen-pound weight loss. For the first time in her life, she had actually dropped pounds without dieting.

A few days later, she began bingeing again. "I'm freaking out," she said. "I can't shove food into my mouth fast enough. What is going on?"

Dawn knew that she was sabotaging herself, but she could not figure out why. If, like Dawn, you're always on a diet but just never quite reach your goal weight, or if you get to a healthy weight but it's impossible to stay there, if you find yourself sabotaging your diet and regaining the weight you lost, then there is a reason. Maybe what you really want, which is to lose weight, is also causing some hidden anxiety. As strange as it may sound, you may be conflicted about changing your body. In this chapter we'll explore some of the fears that may be holding you back from successful, sustainable weight loss.

WHAT IS KEEPING YOU STUCK?

At this point you may be thinking, "That sounds crazy. Of course I want to lose weight. I'm not scared to be skinny." Consciously you likely have lots of good reasons to lose weight. Depending on your situation, those reasons might have to do with your health: eliminating diabetes or sleep apnea; lowering your risk of a heart attack, stroke, or cancer; being less depressed or anxious; walking or running without getting winded; and keeping up with your kids, if you have them. Or the reasons might be about your appearance. You want to wear a bathing suit in public and look at photos of yourself without wincing. Or maybe you're embarrassed to ask for a seat-belt extension on an airplane. Maybe you just want to sit in a restaurant booth without worrying if you're going to fit.

Yes, there are lots of logical reasons to lose weight. But remember, *we are ruled not by the logical, but rather by the psychological.* Often the most powerful influences on our behavior are the thoughts and beliefs that are hidden—they're out of awareness but not out of operation. When you recognize and work through them, you can set yourself free.

What is keeping you stuck? What are these hidden anxieties that prevent you from reaching or remaining at a healthy goal weight? These include fears of success, failure, expectation, impulsivity, objectification, intimacy, and one more that may surprise you.

Fear of Success

The very phrase sounds counterintuitive. Why would anyone be afraid of success? Fear of success can be related to concerns about maintaining success, worries about making other people envious, or feeling unworthy of anything too good.

A lot of people worry that once they're successful they won't be able to maintain their success. If you don't allow yourself to become too happy (or too thin), then you don't have to worry about it being taken away.

One of my patients feared success because she didn't want to make anyone jealous. She and her friends bonded over their failed diets, struggles with weight, and shopping trips to plus-size stores. She worried that once she lost weight, she would lose her friendships too. What would they talk about if they couldn't bond over their shared diet failures and efforts to lose weight? She feared if she was a success story and lost weight, she'd lose her connection to her friends.

Many people fear success because they don't think they deserve anything good, which is usually related to childhood experiences. When children are treated badly, they think they're bad. This "bad" treatment doesn't necessarily have to be outright physical, sexual, or emotional abuse (although it can be), but rather any experience that undermines a child's sense of self, which has a lasting effect.

It's easier for kids to think that their parents or schoolmates are treating them badly because they deserve it than it is for them to believe others can be cruel or dismissive without reason. It's horrific to think you have inept, careless, or anxious parents because that makes the world seem a lot less safe.

If you're the bad one, you also have the illusion of hope. The idea is that if you can figure out what's wrong with you and make yourself good, you'll finally get the parenting or loving treatment that you want. The trouble is that this strategy for giving yourself hope winds up as confirmation of your essential badness. If you think you're bad, then you may not feel as if you deserve to be happy and successful. After all, bad people deserve to be punished, not rewarded. Thinking that you're bad or that there is something wrong with you is a strategy for surviving difficult circumstances in childhood that becomes a conviction about who you are as a person. Believing that you do not deserve success becomes a self-fulfilling prophecy, making it impossible for you to create a healthy, happy relationship with food, stop bingeing or stress eating, and lose weight for good.

Fear of Failure

Fear of failure is related to perfectionism, rejection, and judgment. Many of us feel like failures when we fail to succeed at something. When Nikki experienced a breakup recently, she was upset, but not about the loss of the relationship—she felt she had missed another opportunity to find "the one" and get married. To her it meant that she was a failure at relationships. Although Nikki's relationship had definitely ended, she was not a failure. If, like my patient, you personalize the failures in your life, you will constantly feel bad about yourself. When that happens, the failure becomes a character flaw in your mind instead of a situation that didn't work out. Keep in mind, the "u" in failure isn't spelled Y-O-U.

Most successful people built their success on the steps of failure. Michael Jordan famously said, "I've missed more than 9,000 shots in my career. I've lost almost 300 games. 26 times I've been trusted to take the game winning shot and missed. I've failed over and over and over again in my life. And that is why I succeed."

Steve Jobs was fired from Apple, the company he helped build. He later said getting fired from Apple was the best thing that could have happened to him. As he said, "The heaviness of being successful was replaced by the lightness of being a beginner again," and it freed him "to enter one of the most creative periods" of his life.

Interesting choice of words, don't you think? For him, heaviness had to do with expectation and lightness with possibility.

Oprah Winfrey was fired from her job as a TV reporter and told she was *unfit* for television. Unfit. Good thing she didn't let someone else's opinion of her influence her belief in herself!

For years, Thomas Edison tried to invent the light bulb. He once said, "I have not failed 700 times. I have succeeded in proving that those 700 ways will not work. When I have eliminated the ways that will not work, I will the find the way that will work." And he did.

So if you've been on 700 diets or lost and gained the same 7, 70, 170, or 700 pounds over and over again, you haven't failed. You just haven't found the right way to lose weight.

Fear of Expectation

Jennifer thought the reason she was passed over for a promotion at work was her weight. She said, "They gave the job to the skinny girl. She looks the part, so she got it." This was a corporate job in which appearance was not a factor, but Jennifer was convinced that the only reason she didn't receive the promotion was her weight.

I've heard people say things like, "When I lose weight, I'll finally [fill in the blank—get a boyfriend or a girlfriend, get married, have kids, get a better job, go back to school, and so on]." There's an expectation that once they lose weight, they will absolutely get the job, the boyfriend, the girlfriend, whatever they want.

But what if they're wrong?

Remember Dawn, who freaked out over the seventeen-pound weight loss and couldn't pack on the pounds fast enough? She came to realize that she harbored a deeper fear, which was giving up the fantasy of her Perfect Thin Self.

To reach her goal weight, Dawn had to drop more than one hundred pounds. In her imagination, after losing weight she would be thin, toned, and pretty. Not only that, but she also would be wittier, funnier, smarter, and happier. She feared that the reality of losing weight meant saggy skin, more wrinkles, and less beauty. As long as her ideal weight remained a fantasy, Dawn could hold out hope for a great body, a wonderful boyfriend, and a new life. She was not ready to give up that fantasy for a potentially disappointing reality.

As Dawn said, "What if I lose all this weight and I still don't have a boyfriend? That would suck." Her initial solution to this fear of failing was to sabotage her weight loss and stay at a familiar weight, hanging on to the fantasy of who she could be if she lost weight.

In other words, weight can function as an excuse for not being where you want to be in life. But what if you get to a healthier ideal weight and none of those things happen? Dawn might have to realize that getting a boyfriend takes more than losing weight. Jennifer, the corporate executive, might have to look at other reasons she didn't get the job, and those reasons might be more troubling to her than her weight. If she cannot blame weight for why she was rejected, then she might have to be open to the idea that the rejection had something to do with herself as a person or with her abilities in her job.

Most of all, the fear of expectation means that you're putting a lot of weight (pardon the expression) on the idea that by changing your weight you will change your life. Because what if your life doesn't change? More likely, when you lose weight, everything in your life will remain exactly the same except for the number on the scale and the size of your clothes.

Fear of Impulsivity

Maybe you can relate to Penelope, who lost the same fifteen pounds over and over again. With each diet she showed impressive dedication and willpower, sticking to the meal plan, exercising like she was training for the Olympics, and eventually losing fifteen pounds. The minute she hit her goal weight, which was 130 pounds, she'd celebrate with some ice cream. And the celebration continued until she gained back all the weight, and then the cycle would repeat.

When Penelope first came to see me, she said she wanted to stop sabotaging herself and start having better willpower. She had undeniable willpower, which she proved every time she went on a diet. I told Penelope that her problem wasn't willpower. (It never is.) The problem was Penelope's fear of what would happen if she allowed herself to stay at 130 pounds.

When I first said this, she looked at me as if I had two heads and said that obviously if she could stay at her goal weight she'd be happier and healthier, she could wear her skinny clothes, and life would be great.

We kept talking about it, and one day she blurted out, "I think that if I let myself get thin and stay thin, I'm afraid I'm going to cheat on my husband."

Penelope had gotten married young, never dated much, and now she was thinking about what she might have missed. As long as she carried fifteen extra pounds, she was sure she would not act on her impulses. After all, she reasoned, no one would want to have sex with her while she was overweight. This idea served a purpose to make sure that she never lost weight. By maintaining her weight and making it the main issue in her life, she avoided thinking about her marital problems. It was not until she recognized and worked through the issues in her relationship that she was able to lose weight for good.

Like Penelope, you may be afraid of what you might do if you lose weight. People have told me that they're afraid of leaving their husbands, cheating on their wives, taking risks at work, or prioritizing themselves. I've heard from countless women that they cannot put themselves first because they're overweight, as if the number on the scale renders them second-class citizens. If this resonates with you, the next step is exploring those fears.

One thing you need to know about fears regarding impulsivity is that fears can disguise wishes. For example, Penelope's fear of cheating on her husband actually expressed a wish to cheat on him. Another client's fear of an impulse to return to graduate school, which would have economic consequences on his family, actually was a disguised way of communicating that he wanted to change professions. As long as he was focused on his weight, he didn't get in touch with his professional dissatisfaction. Therefore, whatever you're worried about might hold a clue as to what you really want. When you face the fears, they lose their power.

Fear of Objectification

People who have negative experiences with intimacy are often afraid of being viewed as objects. Whether they were abused or shamed in some way about their appearance or sexuality, they may try to disappear from view by being overweight because that makes them feel invisible. One example is Cynthia, who had a deep fear of male attention and never married or had children. She brought a baby photo into session one day, a picture of herself when she was about a year old, sitting in a bathtub.

"Look at that," she said. "I still have the exact same body I did when I was a baby."

For Cynthia, staying chubby and round like a baby meant looking asexual and nondescript. She often prodded her stomach, exclaiming, "Who would want to touch this? It's gross." Staying at a weight that she labeled as "gross" served to protect her from the possibility of being intimate with a man. She got nervous at the thought of being perceived as sexy. She knew that some men are attracted to bigger women, but she wanted nothing to do with them. Why was she so anxious about physical closeness? As a child, she witnessed her father being verbally abusive to her mother. Her mom was passive and did not defend herself. Cynthia came to associate being in a relationship with being vulnerable to abuse. Logically she knew that all relationships aren't power struggles, but her fear was more powerful than what her mind told her was logical.

Cynthia also had the "pretty face" syndrome. People were always saying that she had "such a pretty face," and if she could just lose weight, guys would be lined up around the block. The truth is, there are guys out there who like curvy, voluptuous, plus-size women. Cynthia could have found someone who liked her just as she was. But she didn't. Why? She was afraid that if she were in a relationship she'd lose her autonomy and dignity, because that's what happened to her mother. As long as she was heavy, she was not at risk of losing herself, or so she believed. Her weight protected her from attention that made her uncomfortable because she connected intimacy with a loss of selfhood.

Cynthia and I processed this belief that her weight kept her safe. She was able to realize this was only an idea she held as a truth, not an actual fact. When she saw that her weight didn't actually serve as protection from male attention, she was able to make healthy choices and eat until she was full but not stuffed. She effortlessly started dropping pounds and didn't regain any weight.

Another client who felt that her weight served to protect her was Donna, who was only ten years old when a neighbor molested her. She began gaining weight shortly after the abuse began, and when she got heavier, her abuser stopped touching her. Donna believed that her weight served as a shield and kept her from being objectified. Now in her thirties, Donna saw losing weight as essentially putting a target on herself. So she stayed big.

Renata had not dated since high school. Her obesity posed a significant health risk, but she refused to lose weight. She also declined to participate in dating websites or apps for men who preferred larger women.

She said, "I don't want a guy to like me because of the way I look. I want him to like me for who I am inside."

I explained to Renata that attraction is based on physical, emotional, and intellectual compatibility. Appearance isn't the only aspect of what draws us to others, but it does matter. If it didn't, we'd all wear burlap sacks and never brush our hair. Renata's fear was that if she lost weight, she would be objectified and used as an object. Her solution was to stay heavy, ensuring that she would not be a "thing" to anyone.

Many years ago I treated an adolescent girl who was morbidly obese. She kept herself in a cocoon of fat and feared losing weight.

As she poignantly said, "Bad things don't happen to fat girls." For her, as with so many women, staying big meant staying safe.

If any of these fears resonate with you, it's important to figure out why you're afraid of sexual or romantic attention. Start working through your associations to intimacy, and to relationships, by considering what you fear will happen if you feel attractive, and why. Often the answers lie in the past, when something bad *did* happen. When people have negative experiences in their childhoods, they often grow into adults who are hypervigilant, always on the lookout to make sure nothing bad ever happens again. Weight can serve as a form of protection, one that imprisons as well as protects. People are viewed as unsafe, and food becomes the only safe refuge.

Fear of Intimacy

If you remember Julia Roberts's character in the film *Runaway Bride*, you'll probably recall that she liked the same kind of eggs as her various fiancés. If a fiancé liked scrambled eggs, she liked scrambled eggs. If he liked them over easy, so did she. She had no idea what kind of eggs she actually preferred.

Similarly, Tonya dated a fireman who loved camping, hiking, mountain biking, and other outdoor activities, so she became an "outdoorsy girl." Her next boyfriend played in a local symphony, and Tonya immersed herself in the world of classical music. In truth, Tonya didn't particularly like either of those activities, but she took them up with great enthusiasm, forgetting her own interests in the process. For Tonya, closeness with another person meant giving up her identity and taking on that of the guy she was with. She gained weight and used her size to avoid meaningful connection.

When you perceive relationships as healthy and associate intimacy with increasing your enjoyment of life, you will not fear connection. When you have fulfilling relationships, you stop seeking companionship (and literal fulfillment) from food.

The last fear that might be keeping you scared to be thinner may surprise you. It is . . .

Fear of Happiness

Don't get me wrong. You don't have to be any particular weight to fully enjoy life and be happy. But if you're putting your life on hold or telling yourself you'll be happier once you lose weight, then maybe you're afraid to be happy. Whenever I mention this as a possibility, people object. They say it doesn't make sense. They tell me they're miserable and uncomfortable. Of course they want to be happy.

"I had such a good weekend," said Cleo, who had recently gotten married. "We went out with friends on Friday night, then we had people over for a barbecue, and I didn't think about food much at all. It was a miracle. Sadly, it was too good to last. The next day my husband went out to play golf and all I did was stay at home and stuff my face with leftovers."

Cleo had a pattern of bingeing on food immediately after experiencing good or happy events in her life. "Maybe you felt like you were just a little too happy," I said. "It could be that you're afraid of happiness."

Cleo made a face. "Are you kidding? Happiness is what it's all about. All I want is to be happy! But as long as I'm eating the whole kitchen, I'm never going to be happy."

Cleo had enjoyed a carefree and happy childhood until her father lost his job and the family's financial circumstances changed. They moved from Connecticut to Florida, and it was like moving to another planet. She didn't fit in and felt uncomfortable. On some level Cleo made a connection between her happy childhood and the subsequent feeling of economic deprivation. Her way of making sure this never happened again was to never allow herself to be too happy. If she never let herself feel too good, that happiness could not be taken away from her. One way she did this was by overeating and worrying about her weight.

Like Cleo, many people are nervous about being happy. They're afraid that if they get too happy, the proverbial rug will be pulled out from under them. They don't allow themselves to become too happy because they're afraid they'll lose their happiness, so they sabotage themselves—as if by daring to be happy, they're inviting punishment from the universe.

Perhaps you attach a positive meaning to unhappiness: True artists must suffer, or it's noble to struggle, or suffering makes you a better person. That could translate into a notion that you're a good person if you suffer and a bad person if you embrace joy. These are ideas that you may have taken as absolute truths. But are they? Where is the nobility in constant suffering? What's wrong with enjoying life, loving and being loved, and being happy? When you allow yourself to trust the idea that happiness can last, you'll allow yourself to get to a weight that you're happy with—and stay there.

WHAT ARE YOUR FEARS?

Which of the seven fears can you most identify with in this chapter? Does that fear sabotage your weight-loss efforts? What can you do to eliminate that fear? Pay attention when you notice this fear surfacing and observe how you respond to it. Does your response have to do with food?

❅ ❅ ❅

Identifying the fears that keep you trapped at a weight you don't like, whether it's a fear of expectation, impulsivity, objectification, happiness, or another fear, is a crucial step to change because when you can challenge these ideas, they lose their grip on you. In the next chapter we'll cover some tools that can help you to stay in the present moment, which will also keep you from self-sabotage and enable you to more fully enjoy your life right now.

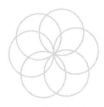

CHAPTER 7

Live in the Moment

"Yesterday is history, tomorrow is a mystery, and today is a gift. That's why they call it the present." I first heard this quote while watching *Kung Fu Panda* with my youngest daughter. To this day it's one of my favorite quotes of all time. Many people imagine the "mystery" of the future in the worst possible way, imagining all kinds of horrible scenarios and feeling anxious about events that have not yet occurred and likely will not happen. That's why it's so important to learn how to stay in the present. Consider the following statements:

- *When I lose weight, then I'll start dating.*
- *When I'm a size four, then I'll be perfect.*
- *When I finish grad school, then my life will be great.*
- *When I get a new job, then I'll be happy.*

Notice the when/then trap that we discussed in chapter 5? When you fall into that trap, you think good things can only be experienced in the future. Think about life as a metaphorical ladder. Are you scrambling to get to the next rung, always trying to get somewhere, to achieve something? If you're always looking to the future, you're never really in the present. If what you want exists only in the future, you never have what you want. Deprivation leads to a sense of emptiness, and feeling empty may cause you to turn toward food as a way of comforting, soothing, or distracting yourself.

Imagine standing on that ladder. Look down the rungs and consider where you started this climb and gauge how far you've come. Remember the growth and change that brought you to this rung of your ladder. Take a moment to appreciate this progress:

- *What were you afraid of back at the bottom rung?*
- *What's different now? How have you changed the way you face those fears or anxieties?*
- *What do you notice about the difference between the past and the present?*

Now think about the rung you're standing upon. Look at yourself, your life, your relationships, and the things about yourself and your life that you appreciate. Take in the moment . . . breathe . . . take measure of your present, both the things you like and those you don't like . . . and hold both.

What do you like about yourself in the here and now? What do you appreciate about yourself and your life?

When you balance appreciating your progress from the past, looking toward the future and what you hope to achieve, with being where you are—in the moment—you'll feel better about yourself and your life. When you feel good you're less likely to turn to food to cope. In this chapter we'll explore how techniques such as self-acceptance, progressive muscle relaxation, visualization, vision boards, and more can all help you to remain grounded in the present.

BE AN OBSERVER IN THE PRESENT

I hear from so many people who are self-conscious about their weight. They don't like eating in public, fearing that other people are judging their food choices or appearance. And they feel this way whether they're ten pounds or one hundred pounds overweight. We feel self-conscious when we think others are looking at us with critical eyes, but the way we see ourselves has a huge impact on how we think other people will see us.

If *you* think you're overweight, unattractive, stupid, or bad in some way, it's easy to imagine that other people are thinking those same things about you. The good news is that the more you develop a positive view of yourself and experience yourself as likable, lovable, smart, interesting, kind, and good, the more likely you are to imagine other people will like you too.

One method to stop feeling self-conscious is to be an *observer* instead of feeling observed. When you're focused on what you see and think, you're less likely to feel under observation.

I once treated a well-known singer who had such terrible stage fright that she would not go on tour. She was certain that the audience was looking at her, judging the size of her body and the quality of her voice, and thinking that she didn't measure up. She imagined that other people were thinking that she weighed more than she should and that they didn't like her because she was heavier than her ideal weight. We came to realize that she had a lot of shame and judgment about her body, which she projected out at the audience and back onto herself.

We addressed her relationship with herself and she became nicer to herself and more accepting. Eventually she felt able to go out on tour again. She called me from Boston, excited to share the news that everything was going well.

"I can feel the energy, and they're really right there with me," she told me in amazement. "They like me."

She went on to tell me that this experience with the audience was so positive that she was certain that new, different people were coming to see her performances. In reality, the fans that were coming to her shows were the same ones who always came to see her. They had not changed, but she had. Now she projected her own self-acceptance onto the audience and back at herself.

BECOME AN OBSERVER

Practice keeping your gaze on the world instead of dodging the scrutiny of others. When you're focused outward, on what you think of other people and situations, and your attention is on them, you're far less likely to feel eyes on you. When that happens, you feel less self-conscious and more at ease. And then you won't turn to food to cope.

SEE YOURSELF WITH MORE CLARITY

"Magic mirror on the wall . . . who's the fairest one of all?" Ever look at yourself in the mirror and think you look okay, even good, but five minutes later your image in the same mirror seems distorted and huge? What you see in the mirror may be reality—or it may reflect an inner conflict.

Our perceptions of our appearance can be influenced by emotions, needs, and wants. If you think you look fat or too big, perhaps that is an expression of your conflict over needs and wants. Do you feel as if you're "too much" for others, or that you want too much? You may imagine that you burden people with your needs. That sense of wanting too much, or needing too much, can be unconsciously experienced as seeing yourself as literally too big.

Similarly, if you grew up in a family in which emotionality was labeled "dramatic" or "oversensitive," you may dismiss your emotions as being too much for others. This sense of being too emotional can then be expressed in concrete physical terms about the size of your body.

Patients often say things like, "I need to lose fifty pounds." They push at parts of their bodies in open disgust, saying, "These thighs have got to go" or "I can't wait to get rid of this flab."

They think that when they lose weight, their lives will improve and they will be more confident, outgoing, and relaxed. (Remember the when/then scenario?) If this sounds familiar, you may believe that by controlling the number on the scale, you can manage many aspects of your life, including your confidence and likability.

Extra weight can also symbolize the qualities you want to get rid of, such as shyness, insecurity, anxiety, and so forth. Losing weight then becomes equivalent to losing those unacceptable parts of yourself. Sure, losing weight may cause you to feel more confident temporarily, but the insecurity usually shifts to something else, such as whether you're smart enough, successful enough, or good enough in some other way. Whereas you once worried about the size of your stomach, now you're concerned about the size of your intellect or bank account. That's why it's essential to address what's undermining your confidence.

When you think about self-acceptance, what "self" do you think of first? If it's the person in the mirror, remember that there is so much more to you than meets the eye. I remember the day I found some of my old journals from high school. As I looked through them, I realized that every page of every journal was about my weight. At the time I thought if I reached some magical number on the scale, then life was going to be perfect. I believed I could change the way I felt about myself by changing my appearance. And I was wrong.

I had to figure out what was eating *at* me, instead of focusing on food. I had to learn that if something's bothering you, you can't starve it away or stuff it down. I had to learn that you cannot measure your true value on a bathroom scale.

I'm fairly confident that no one has ever loved their friends because they're thin and attractive. The thought is utterly absurd. You love your friends because they're nice, they're fun, they make you laugh, and they're supportive, warm, great people.

"Every day, I help people kick the diet habit by making peace with themselves. "

Ultimately, looking in the mirror and liking who you see means accepting the aspects you like about yourself as well as those you don't. Every day I help people kick the diet habit by making peace with themselves. That's the key. Remember, there's a whole range of qualities that make you the unique person you are. There are intellectual, relational, emotional, creative, and spiritual parts of you. It's necessary to identify, embrace, and nurture all those parts of yourself because they all need your attention and appreciation.

CALM YOUR BODY, CALM YOUR MIND

Do you eat when you're stressed? When you're bored, angry, or sad? Maybe you turn to food for soothing and celebration. Even if you're not aware of what's going on emotionally, you might find yourself in front of an open fridge, eating as a way to calm down. Sedating your body with food can sometimes lead to a calmer mind.

Ultimately, of course, you can't eat away feelings, can't think them away, starve them away, or work them away. The only way to get rid of feelings is to feel them. But maybe you're not ready to feel your feelings. Or maybe you just don't want to feel them. If you can't use food for stress relief, how do you relax?

That's the million-dollar question, isn't it?

I'm going to give you some methods to calm your body and your mind—ways that don't involve food. When you're calm and relaxed, you're less likely to use food as a tranquilizer.

Imagine that you're in my office and I tell you, "Just relax."

Does it work? Not so much.

If your mind cannot make your body relax, you need to find a different way to soothe yourself. You'll note that I don't include meditation as one of my methods, and there's a reason for this. Because we often use food to escape our thoughts and feelings, meditation can actually make things worse instead of better. It places us in the very situation we are trying to escape. Many of my patients have tried meditation only to struggle and feel like a failure, and guess what that leads to? A desire to eat for comfort.

One of my favorite relaxation tools is the *progressive muscle relaxation exercise*. You can do this anywhere—in your car, at home, or at work.

Progressive Muscle Relaxation

First, tense up your muscles as tightly as possible. Tighten your legs, then your stomach, and next your arms, thighs, abs, and biceps. Make fists and get your muscles really, really tight, and hold that tension as long as possible. Ideally, you would hold those muscles tight for at least fifteen seconds, but for now let's hold them another 5-4-3-2-1 . . .

Now release your muscles. Completely.

Feel that? You are likely feeling a calming sensation flowing through your muscles. Now that you're feeling a bit calmer, take a deep breath and release it, to deepen the relaxation. When you relax your body, your mind will follow.

The idea behind this exercise is that without muscle tension you can't access muscle release. Create the tension, release it, and enjoy the calming sensation that follows.

The Four Senses

Another way to alleviate stress and anxiety is to stop the escalation of stress. Different people have different responses to stress. Some of us, when we get stressed, become extremely anxious and keyed up. Others get depressed, shut down, and become withdrawn. No matter what your reaction to stress is, you can learn to respond differently.

As you know, our five senses are seeing, hearing, touching, feeling, and tasting. If you turn to food when you're stressed, you're familiar with the sense of taste and use food as your primary method of self-soothing. The *four senses exercise* connects you with the other senses and helps you center yourself.

To help remember the four senses, I like to use the acronym TEEN: Touch, Eyes, Ears, and Nose. Here's what you do: Wherever you are, look around and say one thing that you can touch, one that you can see, one that you can hear, and one that you can smell. Repeat this until you're calmer.

For example, imagine you're in your office. You *touch* your desk. You *see* your computer. You *hear* traffic. You *smell* someone's lingering perfume.

Do it again. You *touch* your phone. You *see* a palm tree swaying in the breeze outside. You *hear* coworkers talking. You *smell* coffee.

Or perhaps you're at home, watching TV, maybe alone or maybe with your family. You're sitting on a couch and you *touch* the fabric, maybe leather or microfiber, maybe wicker. You *see* a picture on the wall. You *hear* a dog barking somewhere. You *smell* a neighbor's dinner cooking.

The more you repeat this, the more you distract your brain from anxiety and the less stressed you will be, which in turn will make you less likely to use food as a coping mechanism.

Visualization

There are two ways to use visualization: One is to create an inner happy place where you feel safe; the other is to practice something you're afraid of. Either way, when you visualize keep in mind those four senses we just talked about.

Think about a place where you feel at peace. This can be somewhere you've been to, somewhere you want to go, or it can be anywhere you can imagine. Maybe you want to be floating in space or living on another planet, or flying your own personal jet pack in the future, or dancing in Paris during the Jazz Age. It's your imagination, so let it take you wherever you want.

Let's imagine you're in Paris during the Roaring Twenties. You're sitting at a sidewalk café, touching your porcelain cup. Picasso is sitting at a nearby table, sketching something on a napkin. Cole Porter music plays in the background. You smell turpentine, probably from the clothes of one of the painters in the café. Relax into this imaginary world.

If that's not your thing, imagine that you're on a beach in Hawaii. You feel the sand beneath your feet. You see endless sky. You hear the crash of the waves against the shore. You hear kids laughing. You smell sunscreen. Whatever image brings you happiness and peace, escape into that image instead of escaping to the fridge. Use your imagination, colored by your senses, to relax.

The second kind of visualization has to do with imagining something that makes you nervous—an upcoming first date, a job interview, or a big presentation. Give yourself an imaginary test run. Practice in your head, keeping those four senses in mind.

Let's use a job interview as an example. Imagine walking into the office where you're having an interview. You shake the hand of the person who is interviewing you, imagining a firm grip. You look around the office, see what's on the walls, what kinds of books the interviewer has, and what family photos sit on the desk. Assess if the office is clean, neat, messy, or comfortable. You hear muted sounds of the air conditioner or the clock ticking. You smell air freshener. You imagine yourself feeling comfortable and confident and relaxed. The more you do this, the less stressed you'll feel— and you'll probably do even better on your actual interview!

How does visualization help you stop bingeing? Visualizing is proactive and reassuring. When you envision a situation in which you are successful, capable, and confident, you're less anxious. Releasing anxiety through visualization means you won't eat for relaxation or distraction. It's an effective way to calm your mind and body so you don't turn to food for that purpose.

Opposite Day

It's easy to get into a rut. You get used to the same things day in and day out. That's why making a new choice can be so powerful. You might choose to change the way you talk to yourself, or you might choose to make a healthy food choice or to do some exercise.

Today you're going to choose something you usually do not choose. If you usually say no to invitations for social gatherings, say yes instead. If you're a social butterfly and your calendar is booked, then say no and spend some time with yourself.

Try making one choice today that is beneficial and nurturing to your body, emotions, or spirit. You'd be surprised at how much making a different choice can affect your life. I know this for a fact because I used to date only tall men. I admit that I'm not proud of this, but I was something of a height snob and I dismissed the idea of dating any man under six feet tall. I dated tons of tall men, and none of those relationships worked out. I decided to date differently and went out with a smart, funny, witty, loving, and generous man who was my height. And guess what? I fell madly in love with him. We've been married for over fifteen years. What's the takeaway from my story? Get out of your rut, do something different, and see how that affects your life. Your life may change dramatically!

Stepping outside your comfort zone often means relating differently to other people. Many of us put on a mask when we relate to people, showing what we consider our best selves to the people around us. We keep our anxieties, fears, and vulnerabilities hidden, fearing rejection or judgment. Since food is a substitute for human connection and relatedness, we turn to food instead of people. Cultivating trust that others can be there for us means we'll have fulfilling, satisfying relationships with people instead of with food.

Another reason it's so important to step out of our comfort zone is because new experiences create a sense of fun, joy, and well-being. When we feel good because we're living fully and authentically, we stop using food for fun, comfort, or escape.

Neutralize Your Fears

Another way to stay present is to categorize the thoughts attached to whatever is stressing you out. Are they thoughts about the future, as in, "What if I screw up the interview? What if I bomb the presentation? What if I come off like an idiot on my date? What if I never feel good enough? What if I never fit into my clothes?"

Future fears can make you have here-and-now worries about something that may or may not ever occur in the future. Recently a friend of mine who had been single for several years after a bitter divorce started to think about dating again. She was freaked out about it. She said, "What if I've forgotten how to flirt? What if I just don't know what to say to guys? What if I'm single for the rest of my life? What if I end up in an apartment with twenty cats?"

Her fears were not likely to happen. I reminded my friend of "what is" to help her gain perspective. When it comes to her fears of flirting, the reality is that she knows how to speak to all kinds of people, in all kinds of situations, and she's never actually gone mute during a date. She's had boyfriends in the past, so it's likely she'll have one again. And she's a dog person, so the cat thing isn't such an issue.

But humor aside, the antidote to future fears is to stay present in the here and now. Also, use the "what if" versus "what is" exercise from the previous chapter to manage your fears and be more realistic. Keep in mind what you know to be true, which will alleviate anxiety and make you less likely to reach for cupcakes when you're stressed.

Although it's important to stay in the present, we cannot help but set goals or think about what we want in the future. Often that gets scary because we feel hopeless and cannot imagine a positive, happy future. That's why it's important to create a specific vision of what you want your life to look like.

Create a Vision of the Future

If you don't have an idea of where you want to be, how will you know when you get there? One way to do that is to create a vision board, a visual depiction of how you want your life to look, a visual that shows what success and happiness look like.

Let's imagine your ideal life. Consider what your day looks like. Think about the people you interact with each day. What is your job? What do you do for fun?

Look through magazines, or a newspaper, and cut out the words and images that appeal to you. Think about what you will feel like, think, have, and do in this ideal life. What new habits will you be incorporating into your life? Create it and watch yourself grow into this new life. Remember, if you can imagine it, you can create it. Creating a vision board is a step toward changing your life.

HOW TO CREATE A VISION BOARD

Step One: Get your supplies. You'll need the following:

- *Poster board (available at FedEx, Rite Aid, CVS, Target, and art supply stores) or a broken-down large cardboard box*

- *Magazines and newspapers*

- *Photos*

- *Scissors*

- *A glue stick*

- *Thumbtacks*

Step Two: Look through all the photos, magazines, and newspapers. Cut out or tear out anything that strikes you— headlines, articles, and anything that grabs your attention. Trust that an intuitive part of you is choosing the right images.

Step Three: Divide everything into categories by theme, such as relationships, career, home, vacation, future, and relaxation. If you have any doubts or reservations about something you picked, put it aside. Again, trust yourself to choose what's right for you.

Step Four: Start gluing! The rule for this step is that there are no rules! Glue everything onto the board in whatever way feels right. Allow yourself to go into a creative zone and feel free to be as whimsical or organized as you want. Optional: Leave a space in the center of the board for a photo of yourself, or just write in your name.

__Step Five:__ Put the vision board where you can see it daily. Ask yourself: What goals am I close to achieving? What goals have I already achieved? What actions am I taking to reach my goal? (And yes, reading this book counts.) Creating a visual depiction of your ideal life helps you clarify your goals, which is the first step toward making those dreams into realities.

Motivate Yourself to Move!

There's a direct correlation between exercise and well-being. Exercise has been shown to decrease both depression and anxiety, reduce stress, and increase self-esteem. Even a small change can yield big results. For example, it may be too daunting to imagine going to the gym or taking a yoga class. But even ten minutes can make a difference. Today, make a commitment to do something physical for ten minutes. That's totally doable, isn't it? Take a walk. Stretch. Do some jumping jacks. Lift some weights. (They can be two pounds or twenty pounds—it doesn't matter.) Put on some music and dance around the house. Whatever form of physical movement you choose, allow yourself to appreciate the strength in your muscles, the beat of your heart, and what it's like to feel truly alive.

Moving is good for your body, and it's good for your soul. Even if you're dancing around the house by yourself, you're going to feel better. I have friends who are always looking for a quick fix to lose ten to twenty pounds fast, and they go from spinning to Cardio Barre to boot camp, to whatever the latest and most brutal form of exercise is, without thinking about whether they actually like it. Then they wind up feeling bad about themselves because they can't stick to anything, so it's always a disaster.

If spinning is your thing, terrific. You're going to get yourself to spin class and reap the benefits of spin class. But if you hate it, don't force yourself—find something you love to do. You'll keep doing it.

I'm a fan of doing something that you like because if you find something you enjoy, you're more likely to do it consistently and make it a lifelong habit rather than force yourself to do something just to lose weight or get in shape. I take figure skating lessons, which is so much fun and so tough, and I also take my 170-pound Great Dane out for power walks. Some may say he takes me for a walk, but either way we're both getting exercise.

One of the regular callers to my radio show is Nick. He used to call in to the show and talk about how he felt lazy. He just couldn't get himself out of the house to take a walk. As it turned out, he was not really a fan of walking. When Nick discovered that he liked to play tennis, he managed to get out of the house without a problem.

Committing to some form of regular movement can help with your weight-loss goals, but not just because you are burning more calories. It can help you release uncomfortable emotions such as anger or sadness that may cause you to turn to food. It can also give you confidence and make you feel good, both of which are important for real and lasting changes.

❀ ❀ ❀

When you relax your body, your mind will follow. When you refocus your mind, you will calm down. When you harness the power of your mind to visualize a peaceful place or use visualization to feel empowered, when you challenge future fears with the present reality, you'll be less anxious. Using these methods to stay in the here and now helps you feel better and be happier. Staying in the present is the last step in your journey to stop bingeing and lose weight. By being in the here and now and learning to respond to yourself in a gentle, soothing way, you'll feel better. When that happens, you won't need to think about using food for comfort or distraction. That's how you liberate yourself from bingeing and live the life of your dreams.

CONCLUSION

Congratulations! You did it! You completed this book and, believe me, that's a major accomplishment. I'm proud of you, and I hope you're also really proud of yourself; it takes courage and dedication to do the things that you've done by reading this book and completing the exercises. It's hard to look inward. It's tough to think painful or upsetting thoughts, feel difficult emotions, and try new things. It's a lot easier to focus on what you're eating than on what's eating *at* you and to break out of your comfort zone.

Let's take a moment to look at what you have achieved. You cracked the code of emotional eating. You learned the real triggers for overeating or bingeing. You started to change your focus—to see yourself and the world in a new way—and you began expressing yourself in words instead of with food.

You also started being a better friend to yourself by encouraging and inspiring yourself. By now you realize that there is so much more to you than the person in the mirror. You've gotten to know yourself better, to appreciate and acknowledge yourself, and I really hope that you have started to let yourself have some fun instead of waiting for the scale to change before you enjoy your life.

I gave you specific guidelines for how to connect with friends and other people, whether they're strangers, coworkers, or family, and a surefire strategy for how to be less nervous and more comfortable in public or at social events.

You started feeding your mind and soul. You stopped the fat talk—that negative voice that makes you feel bad about yourself—and you learned to tame that inner critic. You began taking care of yourself—body, mind, and soul.

Now you have strategies to stop the sabotage that sometimes accompanies weight loss. You also have tools to help you stay grounded in the present. You created a specific vision for your future and clarified the goals that will help you achieve it. You started making new and different choices in various areas of your life to create balance and make that vision a reality.

Although you've reached the end of the book, I'm still here for you. If you haven't already done so, go ahead and join my private Facebook community. The group is called Dr. Nina's "Food for Thought" Community. I'm there to give you information and inspiration; you can connect with others who "get it," and you can find support and motivation.

Thank you from the bottom of my heart for your trust in me and in this book, and for opening your mind and your heart to a new way of thinking about your relationship with food and to yourself.

Now that you have stopped dieting, you can truly start living!

ACKNOWLEDGMENTS

Ever wonder what it's like to win the lottery? I'm lucky enough to have a one-in-a-million family. Writing is a time-consuming, sometimes joyful and other times agonizing, experience. My husband, David, and daughters, Ariel and Kavanna, backed me every step of the way. David reassured me more times than I can count that, yes, I would finish the book, and, yes, it really would help change people's lives. Thank you, my love, my friend, and my partner through life. Hugs to my bright, talented, and spirited daughters, Ariel and Kavanna, for understanding all the long nights I spent at the computer. I couldn't have written this book without your extraordinary support.

I'm thankful for my inspirational mentors, Salman Akhtar and Axel Hoffer, who believed in me when I was about a minute out of graduate school and encouraged me to write. Their guidance and the opportunities they gave me to contribute chapters to their publications inspired me to believe I could write books of my own.

Thank you to Shahrzad Siassi for her unwavering interest, compassion, attention, and kindness. She's taught me that transformation is difficult but possible, and I am forever grateful.

Heartfelt appreciation goes to D.B., whose unexpected friendship and forever sisterhood brought a new dimension to my life, and who occupies a special place in my heart.

Many thanks to my thoughtful and meticulous editor, Lara Asher, whose organizational expertise and thoughtful questions elevated this manuscript to a whole new level.

Ultimately, this book exists because of the many patients and clients who shared their hopes, fears, wishes, and innermost private thoughts. I'm tremendously moved by their willingness to try something new and their confidence and belief in my guidance. It's easier to summon willpower or start a new diet than to journey into the mysterious, hidden places of the psyche, yet each one of them braved that unknown internal territory. Their openness and trust is the soul of this book, and I shall forever be deeply grateful to each of them.

BIBLIOGRAPHY

Bailor, Jonathan. *The Calorie Myth: How to Eat More, Exercise Less, Lose Weight, and Live Better.* New York: HarperCollins, 2014.

Björntorp, P. "Do Stress Reactions Cause Abdominal Obesity and Comorbidities?" *Obesity Reviews* 2 (2001): 73–86.

Blackburn G. L., B. S. Kanders, L. J. Stein, P. T. Lavin, J. Adler, and K. D. Brownell. "Weight Cycling: The Experience of Human Dieters." *American Journal of Clinical Nutrition* 49.5 Suppl (1989): 1105–9.

Buchanan, Kiera, and Jeannie Sheffield. "Why Do Diets Fail?: An Exploration of Dieters' Experiences Using Thematic Analysis." *Journal of Health Psychology* 22.7 (2015): 906–915.

Cozolino, Louis. *The Neuroscience of Human Relationships: Attachment and the Developing Social Brain.* 2nd ed. New York: W. W. Norton & Company, 2014.

Dodes, Lance. *Breaking Addiction: A 7-Step Handbook for Ending Any Addiction.* New York: HarperCollins, 2011.

——. "Compulsion and Addiction." *Journal of the American Psychoanalytic Association* 44.3 (1996): 815–835.

——. *The Heart of Addiction.* New York: HarperCollins, 2002.

Dyer, Dr. Wayne. "I Am a Human Being, Not a Human Doing." Facebook, November 26, 2009, www.facebook.com/drwaynedyer/posts/185464583996. Accessed November 2, 2018.

Ferdman, Roberto A. "The Soda Industry Is Discovering What the Future of Diet Coke Looks Like (and It Isn't Pretty)." *Washington*

Post, March 23, 2015. https://www.washingtonpost.com/news/wonk/wp/2015/03/23/america-has-fallen-out-of-love-with-diet-sodas-and-possibly-for-good/?utm_term=.ce533362de53.

Field, Alison, S. B. Austin, C. B. Taylor, Susan Malspeis, Bernard Rosner, Helaine R. Rockett, Matthew W. Gillman, and Graham A. Colditz. "Relation Between Dieting and Weight Change Among Preadolescents and Adolescents." *Pediatrics* 112 (2003): 900–906.

Fowler, S. P., K. Williams, R. G. Resendez, K. J. Hunt, H. P. Hazuda, and M. P. Stern. "Fueling the Obesity Epidemic? Artificially Sweetened Beverage Use and Long-Term Weight Gain." *Obesity* 16 (2008): 1894–1900.

Gearhardt, A. N., et al. "Preliminary Validation of the Yale Food Addiction Scale." *Appetite* 52 (2009): 430–436.

Greenway, C. M., Loria E. Obarzanek, and D. A. Williamson. "Comparison of Weight-Loss Diets with Different Compositions of Fat, Protein, and Carbohydrates." *New England Journal of Medicine* 360.9 (2009): 859–873.

Hebebrand, Johannes, et al. "'Eating Addiction,' Rather Than 'Food Addiction,' Better Captures Addictive-Like Eating Behavior." *Neuroscience & Biobehavioral Reviews* 47 (2014): 295–306.

Hoffer, Axel, and Daniel Buie. "Helplessness and the Analyst's War Against Feeling It." *The American Journal of Psychoanalysis* 76.1 (2016): 1.

Hutchinson, Marcia G. *Transforming Body Image: Learning to Love the Body You Hate.* Berkeley: The Crossing Press, 1985.

Institute of Health Metrics and Evaluation. "Overweight and Obesity in the United States." http://www.healthdata.org/infographic/overweight-and-obesity-us. Accessed June 4, 2018.

Jackson, S. E., C. Kirschbaum, and A. Steptoe. "Hair Cortisol and Adiposity in a Population-Based Sample of 2,527 Men and Women Aged 54 to 87 Years." *Obesity* 25 (2017): 539–544.

Kinsell, Laurance, Barbara Gunning, George Michaels, James Richardson, Stephen E. Cox, and Calvin Lemon. "Calories Do Count." *Metabolism Clinical and Experimental* 13.3 (1964): 195–204.

Kristeller, J. L., and R. Q. Wolever. "Mindfulness-Based Eating Awareness Training for Treating Binge Eating Disorder: The Conceptual Foundation." *Eating Disorders* 19.1 (2011): 49–61.

Malik, Vasanti S., Matthias B. Schulze, and Frank B. Hu. "Intake of Sugar-Sweetened Beverages and Weight Gain: A Systematic Review." *The American Journal of Clinical Nutrition* 84.2 (2006): 274–288.

Mann, Traci, A. J. Tomiyama, E. Westling, A. M. Lew, B. Samuels, and J. Chatman. "Medicare's Search for Effective Obesity Treatments: Diets Are Not the Answer." *American Psychologist* 62.3 (2007): 220–233.

Mann, Traci. *Secrets from the Eating Lab: The Science of Weight Loss, the Myth of Willpower, and Why You Should Never Diet Again.* New York: HarperCollins, 2015.

Miller, Paige, and Vanessa Perez. "What Do You Say When Your Patients Ask Whether Low-Calorie Sweeteners Help with Weight Management?" *American Journal of Clinical Nutrition* 100 (2014): 739–740.

Murray, Christopher J. L., and Marie Ng. "Nearly One-Third of the World's Population Is Obese or Overweight, New Data Show." http:// www.healthdata.org/news-release/nearly-one-third-world%E2%80%99s-population-obese-or-overweight-new-data-show. Accessed December 19, 2018.

Organization for Economic Co-operation and Development. "Obesity Update 2017." https://www.oecd.org/els/health-systems/Obesity-Update-2017.pdf. Accessed June 4, 2019.

Peeke, Pamela, and George Chrousos. "Hypercortisolism and Obesity." *Annals of the New York Academy of Sciences* 771 (1995): 665–676.

Pietiläinen, K. H., S. E. Saarni, J. Kaprio, and A. Rissanen. "Does Dieting Make You Fat? A Twin Study." *International Journal of Obesity* 36.3 (2011): 456–464.

Popick, Barry. "The Most Dangerous Food Is Wedding Cake." http://
www.barrypopik.com/index.php/new_york_city/entry/the_most_
dangerous_food_is_wedding_cake. Accessed December 18, 2018

Pressman, Peter, Roger A. Clemens, and Heather A. Rodriguez. "Food
Addiction: Clinical Reality or Mythology?" *The American Journal
of Medicine* 128.11 (2015): 1165–1166.

Purcell, Katrina, P. Sumithran, L. A. Prendergast, C. J. Bouniu, E.
Delbridge, and J. Proietto. "The Effect of Rate of Weight Loss on
Long-Term Weight Management: A Randomised Controlled Trial."
The Lancet Diabetes & Endocrinology 2.12 (2014): 954–962.

The Quotations Page. "George Bernard Shaw." http://www.quotation
spage.com/quotes/George_Bernard_Shaw. Accessed September
18, 2018.

Rowling, J. K. Interview with Auslan Cramb. *The Telegraph*. April 6,
2006. http://www.telegraph.co.uk/news/uknews/1514969/
My-daughters-will-have-to-make-their-way-in-this-skinny-obsessed-
world.-Id-rather-they-were-a-thousand-things-before-thin..html.

Sacks, F. M., et al. "Anatomically Distinct Dopamine Release During
Anticipation and Experience of Peak Emotion to Music." *Nature
Neuroscience* 14.2 (2011): 257–262.

Schore, Alan. "Attachment and the Regulation of the Right Brain."
Attachment & Human Development 2 (2010): 23–47.

Smitham, Lora. "Evaluating an Intuitive Eating Program for Binge
Eating Disorder: A Benchmarking Study." Diss. University of Notre
Dame, 2008.

Swithers, S. E. "Artificial Sweeteners Produce the Counterintuitive
Effect of Inducing Metabolic Derangements." *Trends in
Endocrinology and Metabolism* 24.9 (2013): 431–441.

University of Edinburgh. "Eating Is Addictive but Sugar, Fat Are
Not Like Drugs, Study Says." ScienceDaily. www.sciencedaily.com/
releases/2014/09/140909093617.htm. Accessed September 18, 2018.

Volkow, N. D., G. J. Wang, D. Tomasi, and R. D. Baler. "The Addictive Dimensionality of Obesity." Biological Psychiatry 73.9 (2013): 811–8.

Wishnofsky, Max. "Caloric Equivalents of Gained or Lost Weight." *American Journal of Clinical Nutrition* 6.5 (1958): 542–546.

Westwater, Margaret L., Paul C. Fletcher, and Hisham Ziauddeen. "Sugar Addiction: The State of the Science." *European Journal of Nutrition.* 55 Supp 2 (2016): 55–69.

World Obesity: Global Obesity Observatory. https://www.worldobesity data.org. Accessed June 10, 2018.

Yang, Qing. "Gain Weight by 'Going Diet?' Artificial Sweeteners and the Neurobiology of Sugar Cravings." *Yale Journal of Biology and Medicine* 83.2 (2010): 101–108.

Ziauddeen, Hisham, and Paul C. Fletcher. "Is Food Addiction a Valid and Useful Concept?" *Obesity Reviews* 14.1 (2013): 19–28.

Ziauddeen, Hisham, Sadaaf Farooqi, and Paul C. Fletcher. "Obesity and the Brain: How Convincing Is the Addiction Model?" *Nature Reviews Neuroscience* 13.4 (2012): 279–286.

INDEX

ABOUT THE AUTHOR

Dr. Nina Savelle-Rocklin, PsyD, is a psychoanalyst, author, and radio host specializing in the psychology of eating, with a successful clinical practice in Los Angeles. In addition to helping her private patients create a healthier, happier relationship with food and themselves, she hosts *The Dr. Nina Show* on LA Talk Radio. She also offers an online program, Kick the Diet Habit, an interactive action-based course that helps members stop binge eating. She writes an award-winning blog, *Make Peace With Food*, and produces a YouTube video series to help viewers stop binge eating.

Considered a thought leader in the field of eating psychology, she has been featured in *Prevention, Redbook, Real Simple, Shape,* and many more. Her work has also been featured in international press in Britain, Hong Kong, and Dubai. She often appears as a guest on radio shows and podcasts, including *The Dr. Drew Podcast,* and presented at the prestigious American Psychoanalytic Association's National Meeting. She contributed chapters for two scholarly psychoanalytic books, *Mistrust* and *Freud and the Buddha.* Her book *Food for Thought: Perspectives on Eating Disorders* is an Amazon bestseller. She also coedited (with Salman Akhtar) *Beyond the Primal Addiction,* which explores addiction from a psychoanalytic perspective.

Dr. Nina knows that it's possible to completely liberate yourself from problem eating. If there is only one thing you take away from her personal story and professional experience, let it be this: There is always hope.

Made in the USA
Coppell, TX
18 May 2021

55870351R00111